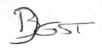 

# The Holistic Guide To Your Health & Wellbeing Today

## A Step-By-Step Guide To The Relationship Between Your Physical, Mental, Energetic & Emotional Health

# The Holistic Guide To Your Health & Wellbeing Today

### A Step-By-Step Guide To The Relationship Between Your Physical, Mental, Energetic & Emotional Health

Oliver Rolfe

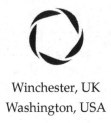

Winchester, UK
Washington, USA

JOHN HUNT PUBLISHING

First published by O-Books, 2022
O-Books is an imprint of John Hunt Publishing Ltd., 3 East St., Alresford,
Hampshire SO24 9EE, UK
office@jhpbooks.com
www.johnhuntpublishing.com
www.o-books.com

For distributor details and how to order please visit the 'Ordering' section on our website.

ISBN: 978 1 78535 392 5
978 1 78535 393 2 (ebook)
Library of Congress Control Number: 2021942472

UK: Printed and bound by CPI Group (UK) Ltd, Croydon, CR0 4YY
Printed in North America by CPI GPS partners

We operate a distinctive and ethical publishing philosophy in
all areas of our business, from our global network of authors to
production and worldwide distribution.

# Contents

# The Holistic Guide To Your Health & Wellbeing Today

*The choices in life are always yours and yours alone. Do not let others define who you are, let YOU define the person you want to become.*

# holistic
/həʊˈlɪstɪk,hɒˈlɪstɪk/
*adjective*

- Philosophy: characterised by the belief that the parts of something are intimately interconnected and explicable only by reference to the whole.
- Medicine: characterised by the treatment of the whole person, taking into account mental and social factors, rather than just the symptoms of a disease.

# today
/təˈdeɪ/
Noun

- in this present time.

# holistic today
/səˈvʌɪvə/təˈdeɪ/

- characterised by the belief that all the elements of a person's health and wellbeing are intimately interconnected and explicable only by reference to the whole, in this present time.

# Acknowledgements

A huge thank you to David Moxon for working alongside me on this journey; it is only the beginning! Thank you to my other partners in positivity…Ann Perry, Sara Leslie, Darren Rolfe and Steps Together (plus Simon, my Natural Health Practitioner). I appreciate all you have done to help put this book together. We are all certainly stronger together!

To my fantastic family, a wonderful and supportive wife, two beautiful children and our dog. Thank you for always trusting and believing in me. I love you all!

To all of you, thank you!

Remembering all those who have lost their lives to the effects of the Coronavirus crisis of 2020/21.

# Introduction

The word 'Gestalt' is a German word and it is very difficult to translate accurately. Arguably, the closest translation we can get to in the English language means 'wholeness' or 'completeness'. This term was adopted by a group of psychologists/philosophers in the 1920s as it neatly summarised their belief in how we should make sense of the world. They called themselves 'Gestaltists' and the three leading exponents of the group were: Max Wertheimer (1880-1943), Kurt Koffka (1886-1941) and Wolfgang Köhler (1887-1967).

Rather than spending time 'breaking' structures down into their constituent parts we need to take a more 'total' or complete view of things.

A useful analogy here is to think of an old-fashioned TV screen made up of thousands of pixels. We could analyse the individual pixels for their colour, activity, intensity etc., however, it is only when we step back a few paces and see the screen completely that we realise each of those individual pixels makes up a recognisable face, person or object.

Seeing the whole picture means far more to us than attempting to analyse each individual component that makes up the image as a whole. In fact, the 'Gestaltists' had a phrase that neatly summarised this idea:

*The whole is greater than the sum of its parts.*

By providing an alternative philosophy to the one accepted by nearly all of modern science, the Gestaltists were attempting to get us to look at things in a different light. Rather than concentrating on individual aspects of life, their argument was to concentrate on the 'bigger picture' first. There is nothing wrong with a detailed analysis of a concept; however, it must first be placed within a much wider context – if we are to make 'true sense' of the idea.

So why start the book with this rather random philosophical idea?

Well first, we believe this 'wholeness' concept is something that has tended to get forgotten in modern times and perhaps it's about time it was resurrected. Our society frequently encourages people to consider elements of themselves, often in isolation. How is your relationship going? How is your exercise regime? Are you eating the right food? How is your physical health? Is there a spiritual element to you? Most of us see them as very important concepts, although understandably struggle to make links between them.

Second, 'seeing the bigger picture' first is how we wish you to think about this publication. Achieving your full potential can only happen if you view all aspects of this process as interconnected.

How you work through your Emotional Intelligence (EI) will be shaped by your physiology, which in turn will be affected by your energy flows at any given time. Achieving some sort of 'synchronicity' between these factors will ultimately affect the person you transform into. Being aware of this 'interconnectedness' (or thinking about the completeness of yourself as the Gestaltists would put it) is a great place to start and finish this book!

We are an integrated system of our physical, mental, energetic and emotional bodies.

*If you can't fly, run. If you can't run, walk.*
*If you can't walk, crawl.*
*No matter what, keep moving.*
Martin Luther King, Jr.

# About the Author

Oliver Rolfe is founder and CEO of Spartan International Group and focuses on life and career guidance and global investment banking recruitment. He studied accounting and finance and started his career with a leading global accounting firm. Oliver then sought a new challenge and moved into the executive search arena in 2003.

In 2003 he began his financial services recruitment career with a subsidiary of S3, one of the largest recruitment companies in Europe. Oliver has spent over 18 successful years specialising in mid- to senior-level individuals with outstanding track records in global equities.

In 2010, Oliver founded Spartan Partnership, and later Spartan International Executive Search, which is a global financial executive search firm. Oliver and Spartan remain focused on assisting those in the markets globally, both on the buy- and sell-sides of the business.

Oliver published his first book, *The Survivor's Guide to Your Career Today*, in 2019 and has been quoted in *The New York Times*, *Bloomberg*, *The Trade News*, *Gulf Times* and many more global publications. Oliver and Spartan have a daily blog that receives over 500,000 individual views a month, over 20,000 followers on LinkedIn, a newsletter/website with over 15,000 subscribers and a YouTube channel – *Spartan Xtra by Spartan International*.

His mission has always been to assist people in becoming the best they can possibly be.

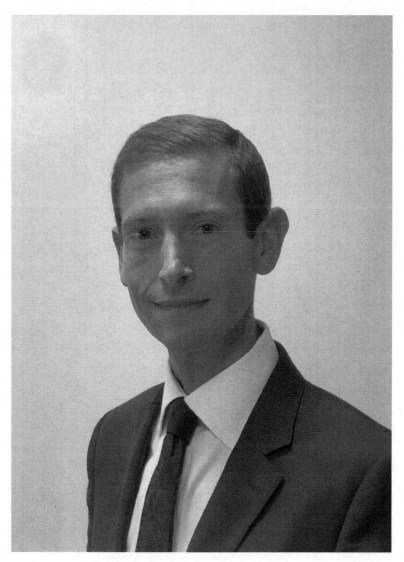

*Picture: Oliver Rolfe*

# About the Editor

David Moxon has spent the last 30 years mentoring and educating people within the fields of health and psychology. He has been module leader for numerous degree programmes as well as supervising third-year dissertations.

As well as running a highly successful private consultancy, he has written three books: *Heinemann Themes in Psychology: Memory*; *Heinemann Themes in Psychology: Human Relationships*; and *Heinemann Psychology for AQA*.

David has also edited a number of series within the field of psychology.

David retired from the academic world in 2020 and now runs a property company and is managing director of Head-a-Head, a specialist outplacement consultancy based in Mayfair.

He has wanted to be involved in a book such as this for some time and thoroughly enjoyed the journey – as Oliver keeps on telling him – NOW is the time!

# We Only Have A Moment In Time

**This is a story of Experience, Understanding and Progression.**

Someone once asked me, why am I doing this? My response is and has always been…to help people. This has always been my WHY, my motivation. This is what I believe we are here for, to help each other. That is how we survive, how we evolve, by helping each other. This is part of our collective consciousness.

By laying bare the very essence of what we have all experienced in life, this can be used and utilised to help many people who feel alone, without knowledge, who do not know that others are going through the same experience, whatever that may be. By speaking out we can ALL win and help each other. The time is now!

While I believe I had a privileged upbringing, none more so than having a loving family and being born in London (UK), I have experienced a number of different life events that made a significant and lasting impression on me. All of these have had a very positive effect on my life and also taught me many important lessons; these include knowing that each experience we have in life comes with its own message or lesson.

For me, these began when I was 5 years old…

My parents divorced, something that a very large number of families go through, especially in the Western world. Due to this, I did not spend a huge amount of time with my father growing up. It was really only at 30, when I had children of my own, that this started to materially change. This time has been great for everyone.

I was fortunate to have a loving mother and grandparents who took the mantle in my early years. My grandfather was an important role model for me, both personally and professionally.

I was extremely lucky and I am eternally thankful to them all.

From around the age of 6 years old to date, I have had over 45 operations, most of which were general anaesthetics, and most at an early age (a major sinus operation at 16 left me with minor nerve damage). As someone heavily involved in sports, I had a few injuries that needed other operations: a broken arm, snapped wrist, knee cartilage, ankle and foot operations. I was surprisingly not accident-prone.

I also suffered with asthma, which made it more difficult to play the sports I loved to be involved in daily. I lost quite a bit of time at school as a result of the operations and recovery time. That said, I was always in either the first or second team for every sport I played (about five), and usually as captain. It was something that happened, and something I always enjoyed.

At the age of 13, I was what you would call...fat, a word I hate to use. I was around 50 pounds heavier than I am now. I was called names, never harshly. I was always sporty, this helped more than anything else. To be fair, I am not sure I really cared until I was about 16, when the other sex became visible. Being big has always stayed with me, and I certainly eat a lot differently now to what I used to do. My family love to remind me of the number of pizzas and hot dogs I ate. What I can say? I like my food. Still do!

Around that time, between the ages of 18-20, I suffered from glandular fever and chronic fatigue syndrome. This was a short time after I had left school and was working for an accountancy firm (BDO Stoy Hayward). I remember having constantly low energy; however, I never over thought it and managed to use my focus on the work to give me the energy I needed. I know that sounds easier said than done; it is! Both glandular fever and chronic fatigue syndrome can be debilitating for many people.

During my upbringing, after the divorce of my parents, my siblings had their own personal difficulties. I remember different parts of these times, and I am delighted to see the strength, drive and passion of them both, as well as the success it has brought to them.

Around the same time that my siblings were going through their own difficulties, I had a difficult relationship with a girl I loved dearly, who was from another country. After nearly 3 years of an intense relationship, we separated and she returned home. It was then that she had told me she had fallen pregnant, with my child (something I never truly believed). Three years later the truth came out and the child was not mine. This was a situation I had to deal with alone at the time. My family was focusing on helping my siblings and I did not want them to have any additional stress. Unfortunately, this had an effect on other relationships around me for some years, until I discovered the truth. As I am sure you can appreciate.

This is something I do not blame anyone for. I have come to realise that we all have our reasons at the time for making certain decisions. We are still learning; we will always be learning.

Moving on…

At 32 I slipped a disc in my back and had to wear a metal brace for 6 months. This made me look like a poor man's Iron Man, rather than anything else. At that time, I was deeply concerned that I would never be able to carry my children or play with them in the park again. That was a tough moment. The only way to get through those situations is to take one day at a time. We can never look too far into the future and be obsessed with what might be. We can only ever affect this present moment. This present moment is the ONLY one that exists.

One small step at a time. One foot in front of another.

More recently, it has been found that I have a total of seven damaged discs throughout my spine and I have been diagnosed with something called Non-Radiographic Ankylosing Spondylitis (an inflammatory disease of the spine). This is most certainly another experience to go through, and something to learn from and assist others with. I am fortunate to be under very good medical care and will continue to progress positively.

While I have detailed some of the struggles that we will all encounter in our lives, and specifically those that I have already ventured through myself, I have failed to mention two life events that could have immediately changed, or shall I say halted, my life forever.

When I was around 3 years old, my family (mum, dad, brother, sister and family friends) and I were out for the day at Regent's Park in London. From what I remember and have in mind, it was a beautiful day and we were so happy being together. We decided that we would all go on one of the rowing boats in the lake, something I had never done before. As the attendant held the boat for us, my dad stepped onto it first, followed by my sister and then me. We were all ready to go, while enjoying the sights of the sunny park, waiting for my mother to get in the boat. As she put her first foot in the boat, for some reason the attendant had let the boat move away from the siding; she was caught somewhere between the side edge and the boat, almost doing the splits. All of a sudden, the boat flipped over and we capsized. From what I was told, my dad managed to get to the side and pull himself out of the water, my sister was able to swim away from the boat, and I...I was stuck underneath the capsized boat. Even now all I can remember is darkness. No sounds, no lights, just pure, black, darkness. I was going to drown! I still have no idea how long I was under the boat, all I do know is that my 7-year-old sister went under the water, and under the boat to find me. Somehow, she managed to grab me and pull me out from under the boat and again from under the water. At that moment, I remember my father grabbing me from my lake-soaked clothes and pulling me out of the water. Had my sister not had the immediate reaction she did, this story could have turned from a dramatic anecdote, to one of tragedy. I am not only fortunate to have a sister who was willing to put herself in harm's way; I am fortunate that there were no forwarding issues, barring the fact that I am not a big fan of going on rowing boats, or many boats as a matter of fact. It also taught me the importance of being a strong swimmer.

We never quite know when our time will be up on the earth plane; however, we have to ensure that we make the most out of every opportunity we have, appreciate all that is around us, and take nothing for granted.

When I was 7 or 8 years old, I had to go through a number of operations. At one time, I had two general anaesthetic operations within 3 months for the same issue. Whenever you have an operation, you are either wheeled down in a bed or wheelchair to the anaesthetist's room, which is connected to the operating theatre, or asked to walk. I always hated walking down, it felt worse. I would always try and calm my nerves whether walking or being wheeled down in a bed; however, I would always arrive with fear. I remember lying in the anaesthetist's room on the operating table, it was always so, so cold in those rooms, it felt like a fridge and usually made my teeth chatter. My mother was next to me, for comfort, as I lay on the table ready to be put to sleep. I never enjoyed that much as a child, as I am sure that you can imagine. The choice of anaesthesia as a child was gas, whereby they used a gas mask, something I also hated. I still remember this so clearly…I really detested the smell and taste of the gas, so I took in the biggest breath I could, and I held it. The issue with holding my breath was that I had taken in a big gulp of the anaesthetic gas, and it was putting me to sleep without me breathing. I remember slipping out of consciousness, that was where the problem started. My mother recalls standing next me, with me apparently asleep, suddenly I started to turn blue. The reality was that I had stopped breathing completely and was now unconscious. She pointed this out to the surgeons who were preparing for my operation. At this point my mother was quickly ushered out of the room before they began to resuscitate me and get me breathing again. Had it not have been for her standing there, who knows what would have happened. I could have suffered a myriad of ills, or worse, not been here to tell the tale.

In the blink of an eye our lives can change and be gone forever. We move through life, especially when we are younger, thinking that we are invincible. We are not. We are fragile beings who may never have the opportunity to fulfil the best of ourselves. I was more than fortunate that someone was looking over me and my family to ensure that I was able to live another day, without any side effects. As a young boy I never understood the gravity of these situations; however, I am still very much here and want to live the best of everyday, especially as I remember and recall these experiences.

**Seize the moment, and do not wait for tomorrow. Make your dreams and aspirations your reality.**

**Take Action Today!**

**This is not a sob story. This is a Success story.**

I would not change a single experience I have been able to journey through. While I would not want to relive those experiences again, each one of them has made me become the person I am today. That is not something I want to change.

**Why am I describing these personal details about me and my life?**

These experiences, mine or yours, do not define who you are in life, they shape you. They shape you into the person you can be and person you can become. You can either choose to be a victim of these experiences or use them to motivate and better yourself, and those around you.

The choices in life are always yours and yours alone. Do not let others define who you are, let YOU define the person you want to become.

**How can this help you?**

This book is the very essence of what I have personally experienced, discussed with many professionals and researched to better understand my holistic self – my body, my mind, my energetic being and my emotional self.

I hope that you can take this knowledge and experience to the betterment of your holistic self.

**Be Positive in everything you do!**

**Take Action Today!**

# It All Starts With You

*The whole is greater than the sum of its parts.* - Gestaltists

# Understanding Your Immune System

With everything that has been happening in the world since the outbreak of COVID-19, it is important, if not imperative, to look after ourselves, and this starts with our bodies and immune system. The immune system is the key to fighting off all infections, viruses and keeping the body healthy. Throughout this chapter we will be looking at the details that make up the immune system, and more so, how to look after and strengthen it. With the help of a number of global health professionals and global data, I have broken these down for you into simple bites.

## What Is The Immune System?

Within our bodies the immune system lives, the protector and defender of all that keeps us well and healthy. Our immune system consists of organs, cells and chemicals, with each one having their own unique ways of warding off and battling microbes (these include bacteria, fungi, algae, parasites and viruses). Should one of these enter the body and a problem arise, our immune system leaps into action and sends an alert signal for our body to release cells. These cells will locate where in the body the attack is happening and will then nullify and kill off the outside intrusion.

The immune system can only do its job and protect our bodies with the assistance of blood, and a liquid call lymph. Lymph is a colourless and clear liquid that passes throughout the tissues within our bodies. There is a total of five litres of blood and lymph that together transport all the elements of the immune system so that it can do its job and protect us.

Apart from being our defender and protector, our immune system has a super-memory that is able to keep a record of every microbe it has ever defeated. This super-memory is recorded in white blood cells, specifically B-lymphocytes and T-lymphocytes. With every microbe being recorded, should the same microbe re-enter our system, it can be quickly identified and destroyed before it has the opportunity to multiply and make us unwell.

Your immune system is your main line of defence for your health. It protects you against disease and infection, and assists with the recovery process after injury or illness.

# The Key Elements Of The Immune System Explained

Our immune systems are constructed with core elements. These include: antibodies, bone marrow, white blood cells, the complement system, the lymphatic system, the spleen and the thymus. These are the key elements of our immune system that actively fight infection and protect us continuously.

## *Antibodies*

Antibodies assist the body in fighting microbes or the toxins (poisons) they produce. The way they do this is by recognising substances called antigens on the outer surface of the microbe, or in the chemicals they produce. This in turn highlights the microbes or toxins as being a threat to us. The antibodies then target these antigens for destruction, which involves many cells, proteins and chemicals in the attack.

Whenever our body is infected with a new antigen our immune system creates new antibodies. Should a familiar antigen infect you for a second time, your body can quickly make copies of the corresponding antibody to destroy it.

## *Bone Marrow*

Bone marrow is an extremely important element of the immune system. Bone marrow is located in the inner core of your bones and is often described as a soft, spongy, gelatinous tissue. Bone marrow contains stem cells that can grow into a various number of cell types. All immune cells come from precursors in the bone marrow and develop into mature cells through a series of changes that can occur in different parts of the body.

The common myeloid progenitor stem cell, located in the bone marrow, is the precursor to innate immune cells. These include: lymphocytes (B-cells and T-cells), basophils, neutrophils, mast cells, monocytes, dendritic cells, eosinophils and macrophages. These immune cells act and respond to infections first and fast.

## Complement System

The complement system is a collection of over 30 proteins that work in unison to assist the role of antibodies. The proteins work together and act like a relay race, where the action of the prior cell will trigger the action of the next protein cell in line, and so on. These actions are usually destroying germs directly or targeting and locating the germs for other cells to seek and destroy.

The complement system works with both acquired and innate immune responses. By locating, targeting and killing germs, the complement system also assists antibodies in doing their job.

## Lymphatic System

The lymphatic system is made up of lymph, a clear and colourless extracellular fluid, and lymphoid organs, which include lymph nodes. The lymphatic system is a network of vessels and tissues, and is used as a method of travel and communication between tissues and the bloodstream.

Immune cells are carried through the lymphatic system and come together in lymph nodes, which are located throughout the body. The lymphatic system manages how our bodies react to bacteria, controls fluid levels in the body, deals with cancer cells and handles cells that would otherwise result in sickness, disease or disorders. The lymphatic system also plays a role in absorbing some of the fats in our diet away from the intestine.

## Spleen

The spleen is an organ in our bodies that is located behind the stomach. The spleen has two crucial roles to play; first it filters our blood by removing microbes and wiping out either old or damaged red blood cells. Second, it creates important elements of the immune system such as antibodies and lymphocytes.

The spleen plays a vital role in creating elements of the immune system that fight off disease and sickness, as well as processing information that it receives from the bloodstream.

## Thymus

The thymus is a small organ located behind your breastbone. The main functions of the thymus include the filtering and monitoring of your blood content, as well as producing white blood cells, which are called T-lymphocytes.

After the cells have formed in your bone marrow, the T-cells then travel to the thymus to develop into cells that are able to identify one antigen from another. At this stage the cells also learn not to self-harm and attack your body's own tissues and good cells.

## White Blood Cells

White blood cells are part of the lymphatic system and play a key role in your immune system. There are two forms of white blood cell, phagocytes and lymphocytes; both are made in your bone marrow.

White blood cells have a short lifespan and will usually only live up to a few weeks. On average, the typical daily production of white blood cells for an adult equates to 10 billion cells, with a single drop of blood containing up to 25,000 white blood cells.

# Simple Steps To Improve Your Immune System – Life Style And Healthy Living

This chapter has been edited with the assistance of Steps Together. Steps Together is a private specialist drug and alcohol rehabilitation group with centres set in tranquil environments.

## Simple Steps To Improve Your Immune System – Life Style

There have been a number of scientific studies since the early 1980s, including that of Dr Dean Ornish, Clinical Professor of Medicine at the University of California, which have proven that with 'lifestyle changes' our bodies can reduce or reverse a multitude of ills, including heart disease. Lifestyle changes include a very low-fat vegetarian diet, meditation/yoga, moderate exercise, stress management and social support. Throughout this chapter we look at areas of our lives we can alter to support and boost our immune system.

### Reduce Stress In Your Life

Stress can have a material and damaging effect on the body, mentally and physically. A vast array of studies have shown that excess stress can harm and weaken our bodies' immune and defence systems.

In times of stress our bodies release hormones from the adrenal gland; these hormones include cortisol, adrenaline and other stress hormones. These hormones work in unison to assist the body in dealing with stress. Under normal circumstances cortisol is useful as it decreases the inflammation in our bodies that has resulted from the immune responses triggered by stress. Should a person be constantly or chronically stressed, then the stress hormones can affect how the body functions over a period of time and can increase the risk of health issues, including heart disease, depression, anxiety, sleep disorders and memory loss.

It is important to find a way to relieve stress in your life; here is a small selection of examples: going for a bike ride, a long walk through nature, meditate, do yoga, talk to a therapist (or close friend), exercise and eat healthily.

## Screens And Screen Time

The average adult will spend around 7 hours a day staring at some form of a digital or electronic screen. This could be a computer, smartphone, tablet, e-book reader, television...even the electronic billboards and signage around town.

Screens play a huge role in our society; however, it is important to limit their use as too much screen time can have a negative physical and mental effect on our bodies.

Research studies, such as those from Dr Satchin Panda, PhD at the Salk Institute, California, have found that when we use screens at night, the red, green and blue light from the screens can affect our circadian rhythms, which can upset and disrupt the process of falling asleep. Our circadian rhythms help us to naturally feel tired and fall asleep as the sun sets, keeping us in sync with our environment. This is why you may find yourself watching a film, reading an e-book or using your computer late into the night without feeling overly tired.

Too much screen time can cause several potential issues, such as eyestrain, blurred vision, short-sightedness, chronic neck, shoulder and back pain, headaches, depression, anxiety, weight gain, insulin resistance and sleep disorders. It can also lead to metabolic syndrome, increasing the risk of type 2 diabetes, stroke and heart disease.

Effectively managing screen time can positively impact our health, relationships and overall wellbeing. Some key tips include; setting time aside for screen-free downtime, not using devices at mealtimes, reading from a book or magazine rather than an e-book or tablet, keeping bedrooms screen-free, spending time outdoors, playing cards or board games, using arts and crafts or cooking. Keep yourself active and free from boredom. Do something you love, and be screen-free!

## *Exercise Is Key*

Exercise promotes healthy living while stimulating your immune system by improving your oxygen levels and blood circulation. Exercise is known to improve our mood and is also a great time to think in our own space, which in turn will help relieve stress.

Exercise, regardless of age, is a key aspect of our lives and life styles. There are many benefits to exercising, whether this is stretching your body, being outside in nature, getting some fresh air, giving you some personal time, improving your mentality, reducing stress etc.

Exercise has many positive effects on your body and it is something you should aim to do every day. When exercising it is important to focus on increasing your heart rate. This can be as simple as a couple of short walks or a long walk every day. You do not have to charge around a sports field to get your heart pumping…thankfully!

While there have been many studies on the effect of exercise on our bodies, it has been found that with regular controlled exercise the chance of developing heart disease decreases, as well as other illnesses such as colds, flu or other coronaviruses.

## *Quit Smoking Tobacco*

Give up smoking! There is nothing positive about smoking tobacco, nothing! (Possibly destressing…come on, seriously?

There must be any number of better ways of destressing than this.)

There are a number of reasons to stop smoking tobacco; most importantly the fact that it is scientifically proven to reduce your lifetime significantly. Of course, there is the social, or anti-social aspect, the smell, the rising costs, the litter, the cost of healthcare, the risk to wildlife…there is nothing positive about smoking tobacco if you value your life.

When you smoke tobacco, you are damaging your immune system and the ability to fight off infections. You are damaging your lung tissue, making you more susceptible to bronchitis and pneumonia. When you smoke tobacco, you are bringing tar and over 4,000 toxins into your lungs; this destroys the antibodies and cells in your body that protect you and aid your recovery from illness. When you smoke tobacco, you are inviting the possibility of diseases such as cancer, autoimmune conditions, respiratory infections, rheumatoid arthritis, gum disease and more.

Quitting this terrible habit is one of the best steps you can take in your life. If cigarettes came out now, they would never be considered for legalisation. Once you quit, make sure you never put another cigarette to your lips again.

## Get A Good Night's Sleep

Sleep is one of the most important practices for our bodies. It is recommended to have between 6 to 8 hours sleep a night. The phrase 'early to bed and early to rise' is very apt here. The more sleep you have the more time you are giving your body to rest, heal and repair. Additionally, as scientific research has proven, for a healthy night's sleep it is imperative that you sleep in a quiet, cool (between 15.6-19.4 degrees Celsius) and completely darkened room, with no light whatsoever.

Sleep deprivation, especially over long periods, is damaging to your body as well as your mental health. Anyone with a child who does not sleep through the night, or is in constant pain, will understand the trials and tribulations of managing daily life with limited sleep; it is not recommended. Get as much sleep as you can, and as you need.

## *Make Love Not War*

Making love has been found to have a positive influence on your immune system. These benefits include: increasing the heart rate, which in turn raises the oxygen levels in your body. The best news of all, the more you do it…the better it can be for you. It is a great time to let your partner know the good news!

## *Keep Clean And Wash Your Hands*

Taking simple steps to avoid infection, making sure you wash your hands with soap and water for at least 20 seconds, singing *Happy Birthday* if you must. It is especially important to wash your hands before eating and after coughing, sneezing and using the bathroom. After all we have experienced throughout 2020/21 with COVID-19, we should all be aware of the importance of washing our hands. It is also possible to use hand sanitiser to kill most germs. If you do so, choose one with at least 60% alcohol, says the FDA and CDC.

## *Spend Time With Family And Friends*

Having strong social connections can have an enormous effect on our health, both mentally and physically. Spending time with our close friends and family lifts our mood and relieves stresses, which in turn is translated throughout your body. Through scientific research, people with healthy relationships have been found to outlive those with poor social ties.

## Cut Out Negative Influences

In life, there are enough challenges to overcome without adding more drama, stress and frustration. It is important to cut out negative influences in your life, this includes those people around you who bring you down rather than lift you up. Whether it is friends, family or colleagues, those who drag you down can effectively suck your energy from you, leaving you in a negative emotional state. Aim to be around people with similar positive mindsets and interests. Those who want to build you up, share in your interests and wish the best for you. It will manifest itself in greater positivity for yourself.

## Meditate And Deep Breathe Regularly

Meditation and deep breathing are important factors in many people's lives. From Buddhist monks, to the most well-known and revered CEOs, celebrities and sportspeople on the planet. A vast number of people feel the benefits and personal development from regular meditation and deep breathing. Further information on meditation and deep breathing can be found in the chapter A Lighter And Brighter You.

## Have A Positive Mindset

It is easy to say 'have a positive mindset'; however, it is not as easy as that to get one. It can take time, training and willpower. Being grateful for what you have and for what you experience is a great way to be positive. The more aware you are of something as simple as a sunrise, or sunset, the more joy and happiness you will experience in your life, and the more positive you will become.

Focus on the positive aspects of life and do not dwell on the negative. Keeping a positive attitude helps your immune

28

system, it will also make you a more likeable person, with more energy to share with others.

## Get Yourself A Pet

On the face of it, having a pet can seem like hard work. They need to be cleaned, fed, exercised, insured and more. That said, giving yourself a reason to exercise is never a bad thing, and the unconditional love and companionship you will receive, especially from a dog, will be well worth the minimal effort a hundred times over.

A study at the University of Minnesota concluded that cat owners were 40% less likely to suffer a fatal heart attack over those people who did not own a cat. Dogs in particular can help a child's immune response and make them less likely to get allergies in later life. Pet owners have been found to have lower blood pressure, lower cholesterol levels, healthier hearts and be less likely to have depression.

## Spend Time With Sun On Your Face

There are many health reasons to get some sun on your face, mentally and physically. For me, the primary reason is to have that warm glowing beam of light on your face, almost filling you up from the inside. The sun does not need to be at its hottest for you to receive its benefits, however; it is said that the early hours of the morning offer the most benefits to our bodies.

Exposing ourselves to direct sunlight helps our bodies produce vitamin D, which has a vast array of benefits for our bodies. Scientific research by the British Association of Dermatologists (BAD) has concluded that vitamin D reduces the risk of bowel cancer, heart disease and other cancers. It has also shown evidence of assisting those with autoimmune disorders and helps you develop good bone health.

While exposure to the sun is beneficial, long exposures can break down vitamin D, reducing the benefit while increasing the risk of skin cancer. The best way to protect yourself and improve your vitamin D intake is to have brief sun exposures, while being careful not to burn and avoiding deliberate tanning.

## *Take Herbs And Vitamin Supplements*

At a certain point in your life, you may feel the need or be required to take vitamin supplements to boost your immune system with what your body is not already receiving from your diet or surroundings (sunlight etc.). The vitamins and supplements you take can range from cod liver oil for your joints, vitamin D to give you the energy of the sun in the winter months or even vitamin C to help your immune system fight off the common cold and winter bugs.

Vitamins and supplements cannot replace a healthy diet; however, vitamins can give you the extra boost you and your body need. In the following chapter we will look at specific vitamin supplements and herbs that proactively assist our immune systems.

# Simple Steps To Improve Your Immune System – Healthy Living

Altering certain aspects of our lives while reducing bad habits and poor routines can have a very positive effect on our mental and physical health, including our immune system. The aspects highlighted below are highly recommended for you to boost your immune system and assist your long-term health.

## *Control Your Coffee Consumption*

The positives and negatives of coffee and caffeine on our bodies have been much debated, discussed and researched globally among science and health professionals alike. The most agreed conclusion is that those who have a particularly high intake of caffeine on a daily basis are likely to experience some ill effects on their body and immune system.

What is too much coffee? It seems that while studies have shown that drinking between 1-2 cups of black coffee everyday reduces the risk of cardiovascular diseases, including strokes, and 4-6 cups of coffee a day could reduce your risk of diabetes by up to 35%, 6 cups or more of either caffeinated or decaffeinated coffee is too much, and could increase your risk of heart disease by up to 22%. Of course, everyone will have their own tolerance levels and it is therefore important to be aware of what your body is telling you.

Too much of anything is not good for you and too much coffee can compromise your immune system by reducing the body's ability to absorb nutrients from your diet, especially iron, calcium and zinc. Additionally, research also shows that drinking a high level of caffeine can lead to stomach upset, abdominal spasms, insomnia, restlessness and panic attacks.

## *Reduce Your Alcohol Intake*

In many societies around the world, alcohol is consumed on a daily basis, with consumption rising over the non-workdays (weekends) and increasing further still with family and friends around times of celebrations. If alcohol had never been legalised and were to be legalised for public consumption in the modern world, there would be outrage and uproar from the medical profession. When consumed in excess, alcohol is a poison to every part of your body.

In a clinical review on the effects of alcohol on the immune system by Dipak Sarkar PhD, Katherine Jung PhD and Joe Wang PhD, they state that it has been long observed that excessive alcohol consumption has an adverse effect on the health of the immune system, which can lead to you being susceptible to illnesses such as pneumonia. This link to ill health has developed further in recent decades with an understanding that excessive alcohol can lead to sepsis, liver disease and cancers. It has also been understood to slow down or lessen a complete recovery from infection, cuts/wounds and physical trauma.

When consuming alcohol is it suggested to limit your daily intake. Men and women are advised not to drink more than 14 units a week on a regular basis (one unit is 10ml of pure alcohol). This is equivalent to six 567ml pints of 4% ABV strength beer or six 175ml glasses of 13.5% ABV strength wine.

While it is important to limit alcohol for health reasons, by limiting your drinking you will save money, you will lose weight (due to the high sugar content in most alcoholic drinks), you will have more energy, be more alert and be a happier person within yourself.

## *Stop Your Intake Of Soft Drinks And Junk Food*

Everyone has heard of the saying 'you are what you eat', and this is no exception. Sugary, man-made soft drinks and junk food offer very little in the way of nourishment and nutrition. Foods such as chocolate, biscuits, breakfast bars, takeaways and fast foods are high in processed fats and sugar, all of which have a negative effect on the immune system.

It is widely known that one can of a regular soft drink has up to eight tablespoons of sugar; that is enough to reduce the active response of your white blood cells to disease and infection.

A study conducted by the University of Bonn showed that takeaways and junk foods can cause an inflammatory reaction in the body, which results in an overactive immune system, alongside changes in our genetic coding. Chronic inflammation on a continuous basis is likely to lead to other health issues such as diabetes, autoimmune conditions and heart disease.

## Eat A Fresh And Healthy Diet

Understanding what we put in our bodies and feed ourselves is vital to our health and wellbeing. This is why having a diet that is high in fruits and vegetables is a great way to give your immune system a boost. The antioxidants and nutrients help your immune system to defend itself and kill off any unwanted infections and diseases. In the following chapter we will look at this in more detail.

## Cut Down On Your Sugar Intake

Eating or drinking too much sugar negatively affects the immune system's ability to ward off bacteria and germs. Sugar can prevent immune cells, which eat and destroy pathogenic germs, from working effectively. This also includes sweeteners, even those that are natural, and refined carbohydrates (bread and pasta).

For a sugar rush with benefits, aim to eat fruits and vegetables that are rich in nutrients like vitamins C and E. They may not have the same taste as a bar of chocolate; however, they can certainly fulfil your sugar craving, while still being beneficial to your immune system.

## *Limit Dairy In Your Diet*

There has long been a debate between the East and West about the use of dairy and cow's milk in our diet. While milk has always been suggested to be a great source of bone-strengthening calcium, it can also have some negative effects on the body. Dairy is known to form mucus in the body which can aggravate the gut. While dairy can affect people differently it is known that it is not something that our human bodies can digest and break down easily. Therefore, it is suggested to limit your intake of dairy and look at dairy-free alternatives such as almond, coconut, oat or soya milk – which are all available in both sweetened and unsweetened versions. I use three of them, depending on what I am eating or drinking. Almond and oak milk usually come out in front for foods, with coconut and almond milk a favourite for drinks, i.e., a café latte or smoothie.

## *Look At Gluten-Free Options*

Over the past 5 years or so gluten-free options have appeared more and more in supermarkets and restaurants globally; however, this is not something new and certainly not a fad. Gluten is a protein that is often found in wheat, barley and rye, and has no essential nutrients. Gluten has been found to cause a reaction (small or large) within a number of people that often results in inflammation and damage to the gut, small intestine and other parts of the body. This reaction reduces the body's ability to absorb virtually all nutrients. Those with celiac disease have an immune reaction that is triggered by eating gluten.

Looking at gluten-free options could benefit you, even if you have the slightest reaction to gluten, such as bloating, diarrhoea, weight loss and abdominal pain. Try eating different pastas made from Edamame (a household go-to), peas, lentils, gluten-free and more, or, instead of breads, try rice cakes or corn crackers. If you are still partial to gluten, rather than white foods, try brown or wholegrain, such as with breads and rice.

## *Be Aware Of The Household Products You Use*

It is likely that you have never thought that your household cleaning products, beauty products and cosmetics could be causing you harm. Within our own homes, on average, it is estimated that there are over 62 harmful toxins we absorb through the air and on our skin. While most of us want to kill off all germs and bacteria in our homes, it is important to realise the negative effects we are having on our bodies and immune systems in the long term. To help protect ourselves we should aim to use cleaning products that have natural and non-harmful ingredients. Using them in a ventilated space, while wearing protective gloves.

The same thought process should be applied to other household products including toothpastes, shampoos, deodorants, shower gels and soaps. Before you use these products, make sure you are aware of the contents and potential negative effects they can have on your immune system, including: Sodium Lauryl Sulfate (SLS), which is a harsh synthetic detergent that can cause skin, eye and lung irritation, Sodium Laureth Sulfate (SLES), which is a milder form of SLS, and Parabens, which are a group of chemicals widely used in cosmetics and are believed to disrupt hormone function by mimicking oestrogen.

## *Detox Your Liver And Kidneys*

Detox is usually something that most people only do after a long weekend, week or month of drinking alcohol and feel the need to replenish and help their bodies recover. This detox is not too dissimilar; however, there is less drinking involved to start with. A detox for your liver and kidneys helps remove excess waste and hydrates the organs.

There are a number of ways to detox, these include drinking lemon or organic apple cider vinegar in warm water, or drinking stinging nettle, hydrangea and sambong teas. Other ways in which you can detox include eating grapes, peanuts, garlic, cilantro, watermelon, avocado, turmeric, apples, spinach and taking dietary supplements.

## *Take Liver And Kidney Supplements*

Looking after your vital organs is key to a strong immune system. The kidneys and liver are no exception and play a vital role in the efficiency and effectiveness of the immune system. While we discuss vitamins and supplements in greater detail in the chapter below, taking vitamins C and B12, curcumin and dandelion tea (or extract) will give your liver and kidneys the additional nutrition and boost they need to function effectively. Wholefood iron vitamins, often combined with vitamin C, are another positivity booster for your liver.

## *Go For A Colonic*

While this may not be for everyone, scientific studies suggest that a colonic irrigation can induce lymphocyte transmigration from lymphatic tissues in your gut into the circulation; this stimulation can improve colon and immune system function.

A colonic irrigation is often used to clear a build-up of toxins in the gut. Many healthcare professionals understand that toxins in your gut can contribute to a number of health issues. From their experiences they have seen that a colonic cleansing has the ability to improve health. This is done by clearing toxins in your gastronomic system and strengthening your immune system.

## Use Epsom Salt

If you have ever had one of those days when your muscles are sore, your bones hurt and your body aches, a nice long, hot bath (bubbles optional) will go a long way to curing your ills. One way to add an additional health boost is with the inclusion of Epsom salt in your bath. The bath will help soothe your body and the Epsom salt will begin to pull the toxins from your body, assisting your immune system. Epsom salt, and the soaking in, increases white blood cells, which fight off viruses and infections. The addition of Epson salt also helps to relax the muscles in the body, relieve constipation, reduce swelling and promote restful sleep.

## Go For A Sauna

It is first important to recognise that health benefits can come from both a traditional and infrared sauna. Saunas by nature raise the core body temperature, which in turn helps draw toxins out of the body, such as bisphenol A (BPA), phthalates, arsenic, lead and mercury. Removing these toxins from the body increases the immune system's ability to work effectively.

Scientific evidence has shown that with regular use of a sauna, the risk of vascular problems such as heart attacks, cardiovascular disease, strokes and high blood pressure drops by 37%. Saunas are also said to reduce stress, help with the common cold and reduce the risk of getting dementia and Alzheimer's by up to 60%.

## *Dry Brush Your Skin*

With many similarities to a sauna, the main reason to dry brush is to remove impurities and toxins from your bodily system. Dry brushing helps to stimulate the tissues under the skin (within the lymphatic system) to eradicate toxins and any unwanted poisons. It is also believed that the dry brushing of glutenous areas can assist with cellulite as it helps the trapped toxins in the fat cells be flushed out through the lymphatic system.

## *Drink Plenty Of Water And Herbal Tea*

Drinking water, or any other non-caffeinated, non-sugary or non-alcoholic fluids, daily is essential to ensure the body and immune system work properly. With a lack of fluids our bodies will not function as they should and will become dehydrated. Keeping hydrated assists the body in fighting infection, especially with hot drinks, sending bacteria to the gut where the acid will destroy it.

The recommended daily fluid intake is 1.2 litres a day, which equates to roughly 6 to 8 glasses of water or herbal tea. Drinking caffeinated, sugary and alcoholic drinks do not count towards the recommended intake. In fact, when drinking those drinks, it is recommended to drink the equivalent amount of water to counteract the negative effects. Keeping hydrated helps the body to naturally flush out bacteria and toxins that could potentially cause illness.

# Simple Steps To Improve Your Immune System – Food, Vitamins And Herbs

## Gut Health – Boost Your Immune System And Avoid Getting Sick

It has long been known that what we feed our bodies has an effect on our health. Our gut health is said to be one of the most crucial elements when looking at the immune system. French scientist Antoine Béchamp, who is best known for breakthroughs in applied organic chemistry, believed that disease develops from within the body due to an acidic and poorly oxygenated 'terrain' (the body's internal environment), and not from external elements. Béchamp's focused work was called the Terrain theory.

Béchamp's theory was initially cast aside by many of his peers; however, with the advancement of technology and years of research the Terrain theory highlights that microorganisms such as bacteria, viruses or fungi are a regular occurrence in the bloodstream, and often cause little or no symptoms of illness. These microorganisms can lie idle and undetected within the tissues of the body for many years, waiting for their activation. Should the immune system become weakened, it is then susceptible and open to attack from these microorganisms. Without an alert and proactive immune system, the microorganisms are awakened and start to multiply, soon overwhelming the body's weakened defences.

Béchamp believed that a healthy terrain (gut) is something that is obtained not only with a nutritious and healthy diet, it is obtained by a healthy and nutritious lifestyle. This includes plenty of fresh air, exercise, mindfulness, good hygiene practices and more. This is about an integrative view of health and being healthy.

Béchamp's theory concludes that a person with a healthy terrain will be largely unaffected by the microorganisms, including germs, that can manifest into diseases within the body, while someone with a terrain that has not been cared for is more likely to be susceptible to infections and viruses.

## The Importance Of Gut Health

It may be difficult to believe, however, nearly 70% of your immune system is located in your gut. Yes, your gut! Due to this fact, it is vitally important to practise and promote excellent gut health.

The lymphoid tissue in your gut is home to immune system cells (leucocytes, macrophages and lymphocytes) that fight and protect your body from viruses and infection. Someone with an unhealthy gastrointestinal system or poor gut health is likely to have a weakened immune system, which can lead to a variety of diseases and illnesses, including infections, inflammation and autoimmune conditions.

# Simple Steps To Improve Your Immune System – Food

## Immune-Boosting Foods

There are many foods globally that will have their own positive impact on our bodies and immune systems. In this chapter we specifically take a closer look at those foods that are immune-boosting foods and those that really give our systems the extra oomph we sometimes need. In general, it is important to have a full and varied diet full of nutritious vitamin enhancing fresh vegetables and fruits, quality proteins and healthy fats. All nutrient data has been confirmed by the USDA National Nutrient Database for Standard Reference, Release 21 (USDA SR-21).

### *Avocado*

This wonderful fruit has come to the Western world's attention quite recently, usually served over speciality breads with an egg, a crack of black pepper and chilli. Avocados are packed with immune-boosting vitamins such as vitamins A, E, C, K and B6, as well as being an excellent source of folate, lutein, magnesium, potassium, glutathione and more. Glutathione is a powerful antioxidant capable of preventing damage to important cells. As an additional advantage, unlike most fruits, avocados have a very low sugar content.

According to a study on hass avocados and potential health effects by Mark L. Dreher and Adrienne J. Davenport (and eight subsequent studies), consuming avocados is said to support weight management, blood glucose control, healthy ageing and have demonstrated positive effects on cardiovascular health.

## *Berries (blueberries, cranberries, raspberries, strawberries)*

Fresh fruit provides our bodies with an abundance of health benefits, and berries are no different. Berries such as blueberries, blackberries, cherries, raspberries, strawberries etc. provide a great source of antioxidants, vitamins C, D and K1, fibre, magnesium, potassium, folate, iron and more.

Through scientific studies, dark berries such as blueberries, blackberries and raspberries have been found to have the highest levels of antioxidants. Berries have also been found to have anti-inflammatory properties, help lower cholesterol, lower blood pressure, improve skin health, protect against cancers and can help keep your heart healthy.

## *Black Tea, Green Tea And Matcha*

First, what is matcha? Matcha is made from dried young green tea leaves by grinding them into a fine powder. To drink matcha, once in powder form, 3-5 teaspoons are placed into a cup of boiling water and stirred thoroughly (putting the matcha through a sieve can help remove lumps). Matcha can be used in ice cream, smoothies, cakes, etc. and has amazing immune-boosting effects.

Matcha and green tea contains a high content of the catechin antioxidant called EGCg (7380mg per 100g), while black tea contains a lesser amount (936mg per 100g). EGCg is an incredible defence for your immune system, defending it against viruses and bacteria, as well as stopping the development of many microorganisms that cause disease. These include the herpes virus, influenza A and hepatitis. EGCg has been proven to reduce inflammation, improve gut health, help with weight loss, lower blood sugar levels and reduce the risk of brain and heart disease.

While ingesting matcha, green tea and black tea can have a positive effect on your immune system, it is important to be aware of the caffeine content, and limit your intake where necessary. One cup of matcha, made with 4 teaspoons of powder, can have up to 280mg of caffeine, whereas a cup of black tea can contain up to 47mg of caffeine.

## Broccoli, Brussels Sprouts, Cabbage, Cauliflower – all the brassicas are excellent

The brassicas, or cruciferous, vegetable family include the likes of kale, broccoli, cauliflower, kohlrabi, cabbage, brussels sprouts and more. These earthy, and often dark green, vegetables are rich in antioxidants, vitamins C and E, folic acid and minerals such as iron, potassium and selenium – all giving the immune system a boost.

A study on the effects of brassica vegetables on human health by the Department of Human Nutrition, Agricultural University of Cracow, led by Joanna Kapusta-Duch, suggests that brassica vegetables' health benefits have been linked to phytochemicals. Phytochemicals have been known to increase the functionality of the immune system, reduce oxidative stress, inhibit carcinogenic mutations and decrease the risk of cancers (prostate, lung, breast and colon).

## Carrots

Ever since Bugs Bunny (with carrot in hand) said, 'What's up Doc?' in the film *A Wild Hare* in 1940, carrots have been a staple root vegetable in households and restaurants across the globe. We have been told for generations that carrots help us see in the dark; can that be true? Carrots are a rich source of beta-carotene (a compound that keeps our eyes healthy) and vitamin A. Both play an important role in assisting our eyes to convert light into a message for our brain. When there is low light or it is dark, it helps us to receive and transmit more light to the brain, improving night vision.

As well as being a rich source of beta-carotene and vitamin A, carrots also offer lower levels of vitamins K and C, as well as potassium, fibre, antioxidants, calcium and iron. Which means, as well as improving your eyesight, carrots also boost the immune system, lower the risk of cancer, help with constipation and keep the heart healthy.

## Citrus Fruit (lemons, grapefruit, oranges)

Apart from being some of the tastiest and zestiest fruits on the planet, citrus fruits offer an array of positive effects for your body. Citrus fruits are known for being a great source of vitamin C, they also boast good amounts of magnesium, flavonoids, fibre, potassium, and A and B6 vitamins. These vitamins and nutrients help boost the immune system and can protect the body against numerous conditions such as diabetes, heart and brain disease, cancer and kidney stones.

It is suggested that you eat whole fruits rather than drink processed juices, due to the addition of vast quantities of sugar. Eating or drinking the most natural ingredients, either from the ground or tree, will ensure your body is receiving as many nutrients as possible for your immune system to benefit.

## Garlic

Garlic has been hailed all over the world as a hero for health, not to mention protection from vampires. A single clove of garlic contains up to 12mg of potassium, 5mg of calcium and over 100 sulfuric compounds, which are strong enough to destroy bacteria and infections.

Garlic has been used throughout history for health reasons in many different guises. Richard S. Rivlin, from the Department of Medicine, Memorial Sloan-Kettering Cancer Center and

Weill Medical College of Cornell University, New York, wrote in *The Journal of Nutrition* that Greek physician Hippocrates prescribed garlic for treating respiratory problems, parasites, digestion issues and fatigue. Nowadays we know that garlic reduces inflammation, improves cardiovascular health, boosts immunity, helps lower cholesterol and reduces the risk of lung, prostate, breast, stomach, rectal and colon cancer.

A study published in the journal *Food and Chemical Toxicology* by the Department of Physiology and Institute of Health Sciences, Gyeongsang National University School of Medicine found that heating garlic reduces its anti-inflammatory effects. They concluded that raw garlic offers the most health benefits. Due to garlic being highly pungent and challenging to eat raw, many people often prefer taking a garlic supplement.

## Ginger

Ginger can be a bit of an acquired taste, especially when eaten in raw form, as it can have quite a kick. Ginger is used to help digestion, fight colds and flu, reduce nausea and inflammation, support cardiovascular health and lower the risk of cancer. Ginger contains high levels of Gingerol, which is the main bioactive compound of ginger. According to research, Gingerol has strong anti-oxidising and anti-inflammatory effects, which boost immune health.

Introducing, or increasing, foods and drinks that include natural ginger will reduce inflammation in your body, keep your immune system healthy and protect you from coughs, colds and flu.

## Kiwi Fruit

Kiwis are packed with nutritious goodness and are full of nutrients such as vitamins C, K, E, potassium, iron and folate.

Additionally, kiwis have a lot of antioxidants and are a good source of fibre. One cup of kiwi amounts to 273% of the daily recommended allowance of vitamin C (nutrient data by the USDA SR-21).

Due to their antioxidants and immune-boosting effects, kiwis are said to promote positive heart health, lower blood pressure, aid digestion, help with sleep disorders and even treat asthma.

## Leafy Green Vegetables (chard, kale, spinach)

Similar to the brassicas above, dark, leafy green vegetables are a fantastic source of vitamins A, C, E, K, and many of the B vitamins. Dark leafy greens also contain high levels of iron, folate, antioxidants, fibre, potassium and calcium, making these a must to include in your daily diet.

Leafy greens can have a huge impact on the body, from the nutritional benefits of the vitamins and minerals, to the health benefits such as lowering the risk of cancers, protecting bone health, preventing inflammatory diseases and supporting the immune system, especially gut health.

Kale, spinach, microgreens and collard greens are said to contain the highest levels of nutrients. According to nutrient data by the USDA SR-21, one cup of raw kale provides 684% of the recommended daily allowance (RDA) of vitamin K, 206% of the RDA of vitamin A and 134% of the RDA of vitamin C.

## Mushrooms (especially oyster and shiitake mushrooms)

Mushrooms are usually classified as a vegetable; however, all mushrooms are in fact fungi. It is therefore important to know what you are ingesting beforehand, as many wild species can be poisonous.

Mushrooms have plenty of health benefits and are full of antioxidants, copper, potassium and B vitamins. One cup of shiitake mushrooms contains 65% of the RDA of copper, 52% of the RDA of vitamin B and 51% of the RDA of selenium. One cup of raw oyster mushrooms boasts 37% of the RDA of vitamin B3, 30% of the RDA of vitamin B2 and 18% of the RDA of phosphorus, potassium and copper (nutrient data by the USDA SR-21).

Due to mushrooms' high content of vitamins, minerals and antioxidants, they have the ability to assist the body in reducing blood pressure, aiding weight loss, reducing the risk of cancers, boosting the immune system and promoting a healthy heart. The most effective way to receive the medicinal benefits of mushrooms is to consume them in dried powder form, rather than in cooking.

## *Salmon*

Salmon has long been considered an immune-boosting food, largely due to the abundance of omega-3 fatty acids, B vitamins (B3, B6, B12), vitamin D, protein, selenium and more. Salmon is an amazing source of nutrients and proteins for the body.

Omega-3 fatty acids play an important role in the body, even if they are not produced by the body itself. Research studies on the effects of Omega-3 on the body have found that it can lower the chances of cardiovascular disease, dementia, inflammation and cancers. It also has a positive effect on your eyes, skin, joints and aids brain function. The high levels of vitamin B12 assist cognitive function, reduce blood pressure and boost the immune system, specifically helping the blood and nerve cells.

According to an environmental health study in 2010 led by Arnold Schecter from the University of Texas School of Public Health, it is important to be aware that salmon was found to be one of the most contaminated fish with hexachlorobenzene (a fungicide that has been banned globally due to the negative effects on the nervous system) and polychlorinated biphenyls or PCBs (industrial products or chemicals that have been shown to affect the immune, nervous and reproductive systems and cause cancer in animals).

## Sweet Red Peppers

Red peppers are full of nutrients that boost the immune system, as well as providing other health benefits. They are a rich source of vitamins A, C, B6 and K, and also provide the body with potassium, folate and fibre.

Green sweet peppers contain over 200% of the RDA for vitamin C, whereby red sweet peppers contain an amazing 317% of the RDA for vitamin C (per a 149g serving). These sweet peppers are able to boost the immune system while assisting the body to maintain healthy skin and vision, and reduce the risk of anaemia, arthritis and cancers (colon, stomach, mouth, throat and lungs). Nutrient data by the USDA SR-21.

## Sunflower Seeds, Almonds And Nuts

Nuts and seeds are eaten by so many of the animal kingdom; this includes smaller animals such as rodents, birds, squirrels, monkeys, as well as larger animals including deer, black bears and elephants. The reason for this is due to their high levels of vitamins, minerals and proteins, not to mention the taste!

Sunflower seeds are an amazing source of vitamins E, B5, B9, phosphorus, selenium, manganese, copper and protein, whereas almonds provide high levels of vitamins E and B2, magnesium, selenium, copper, phosphorus, protein and fibre. Other nuts and seeds that are good sources of nutrition include: cashews, chia seeds, flaxseeds, hemp seeds, pecans, walnuts, pistachios and Brazil nuts.

There is mounting scientific evidence to suggest that eating seeds and nuts on a daily basis is good for your health and can lower the risk of heart disease and diabetes. In 2013 at the Harvard T.H. Chan School of Public Health, Dr Heather Baer, Dr Robert Glynn, Dr Frank Hu and Co. conducted a study using 50,112 participants. By analysing multiple risk factors for mortality, including the effects of alcohol consumption, smoking, diet and lifestyle, they concluded that those who ate one or two handfuls of nuts a day were less likely to die from heart disease, cancer or respiratory diseases. The study also suggested that eating nuts can increase your lifespan by 20%.

## *Microorganism – Probiotics*

While bacteria are often thought of as something harmful, there are many bacteria and microorganisms that are in fact good for your body, especially in your gut. These 'good' bacteria help the body to digest food, destroy disease-causing cells and produce vitamins.

Probiotics are live microorganisms that when consumed assist the body in a number of positive processes. Probiotics work to assist the body in restoring gut microflora; this is heightened when there is an overgrowth of bad bacteria, which contributes in assisting to boost the immune system function. Probiotics are also said to have other positive impacts on our health, including improving irritable bowel syndrome (IBS), reducing the risk or severity of antibiotic-associated diarrhoea and other diarrhoea-related illnesses.

Probiotics can be found in specific foods, which include: fermented foods (kimchi, kombucha, sauerkraut, kefir), yogurts and dietary supplements. They can also be found in some beauty products. These probiotic products contain the same, or similar, microorganisms to those that live naturally in our bodies.

# Simple Steps To Improve Your Immune System – Vitamins

### Give Me An A, Give Me A C, Give Me A Vitamin D!!!

Our bodies require an array of nutrients to work harmoniously, with both vitamins and minerals playing a vital part. Throughout this chapter we assess how each essential vitamin and mineral assists our body function, how we can increase our natural intake and what is the RDA.

### *Vitamin A*

Vitamin A is an essential vitamin that plays a vital health role. It assists your immune system against infection and disease, helps your vision in low light, lowers the risk of cancer and contributes to the growth of all bodily tissues, including skin and hair.

Vitamin A is an antioxidant and can come from a variety of food and drink produce such as carrots, avocado, sweet potato, dark leafy greens, eggs, cheese, oily fish and liver. It is also available as a supplement and can be found in most multivitamin-mineral supplements.

The National Institutes of Health (NIH) in the USA suggests:

- An adult male (19+) requires 900mcg of vitamin A daily
- An adult female (19+) requires 700mcg of vitamin A daily

The National Health Service (NHS) in the UK suggests:

- An adult male (age 19-64) requires 700mcg of vitamin A daily

- An adult female (19-64) requires 600mcg of vitamin A daily

## Vitamin B12

Vitamin B12 is an important vitamin for the health of your immune system and your body. Vitamin B12 is needed for the body to make red blood cells, keep the nervous system healthy, help prevent anaemia and convert digested food into the energy you need to function.

As vitamin B12 is a water-soluble vitamin, it means that your body does not keep storage of the vitamin; therefore, it needs to be replenished daily, either by your diet or supplements. Vitamin B12 can be found in beef, liver, clams, meat, poultry, fish and pork. It is not found naturally in plant-based foods, and it is therefore recommended that vegetarians and vegans take vitamin B12 supplements to boost their intake.

The NIH in the USA suggests:

- An adult (19+) requires 2.4mcg of vitamin B12 daily

The NHS in the UK suggests:

- An adult (19+) requires 1.5mcg of vitamin B12 daily

## Vitamin C

Vitamin C is possibly one of the most well-known of all the vitamins available. Vitamin C is an antioxidant and is important for the health of your immune system and body. Without enough vitamin C you could end up with anaemia, infections and wounds or cuts not healing properly. Vitamin C has also been found to prevent cancers and reduce the risk of cardiovascular disease.

Vitamin C is a water-soluble vitamin, like vitamin B12, and needs to be replenished daily. Fortunately, vitamin C can be included in your daily diet fairly easily as it mainly comes from fruits and vegetables. These include: citrus fruits, tomatoes, sweet red peppers, strawberries, blackcurrants, leafy greens and brassicas. It is also available as a supplement and can be found in most multivitamin-mineral supplements.

The NIH in the USA suggests:

- An adult male (19+) requires 90mg of vitamin C daily
- An adult female (19+) requires 75mg of vitamin C daily

The NHS in the UK suggests:

- An adult (aged 19-64) requires 40mg of vitamin C daily

It is possible that the dosage can be increased when you are unwell or have a cold. The maximum daily limit is said to be 2000mg. Too much vitamin C can cause an upset stomach.

## *Vitamin D*

Vitamin D is most recognised for coming from sunshine. Our bodies produce vitamin D when outside in direct sunlight and, in the United Kingdom, we receive enough vitamin D from the sun alone between the months of April and September. Vitamin D can also be found in a range of different foods; these include salmon, tuna (fatty fish), cod liver oil, beef liver, cheese, egg yolks, milk and flaxseeds. It is also available as a supplement and can be found in most multivitamin-mineral supplements.

Vitamin D is a fat-soluble vitamin. Fat-soluble vitamins, such as vitamins A, D, E and K, are an important element within our bodies. These vitamins assist a number of physiological processes such as bone, muscle, vision and teeth health, as well as immune-system health. Vitamin D plays a pivotal role in defending the immune system from infection and reducing inflammation.

The NIH in the USA suggests:

- An adult (19-70) requires 15mcg or 600 IU of vitamin D daily
- An adult (70+) requires 20mcg or 800 IU of vitamin D daily

The NHS in the UK suggests:

- An adult (19+) requires 10mcg or 400 IU of vitamin D daily

### *Vitamin E*

Vitamin E is another power vitamin that assists the body by maintaining eye and skin health, provides a natural boost to the immune system and plays an instrumental role in the formation of red blood cells.

Vitamin E, like A, D and K, is a fat-soluble vitamin, which means it is able to be dissolved in fats and oils. Vitamin E can be found in a lot of differing food groups, including rapeseed, vegetable, sunflower, soya, corn and olive oil, meats, poultry, fruits, vegetables, nuts, seeds, cereals and more. It is also available as a supplement and can be found in most multivitamin-mineral supplements.

Should the body have enough Vitamin E in its system currently, the remaining vitamin E is stored for future use in the body's fatty tissue. Therefore, you should be able to receive all the vitamin E you require from your diet, even if you do not eat foods that are rich in vitamin E daily.

The NIH in the USA suggests:

- An adult (19+) requires 15mg of vitamin E daily

The NHS in the UK suggests:

- An adult male (19+) requires 4mg of vitamin E daily
- An adult female (19+) requires 3mg of vitamin E daily

## *Vitamin K*

Vitamin K (K1 and K2) is an important nutrient that is needed for the body to stay healthy. Vitamin K is vital for blood clotting and ensuring that our bones stay healthy.

Vitamin K, like A, D and E, is a fat-soluble vitamin, which means it is able to be dissolved in fats and oils. Vitamin K is found naturally in many food groups, including green leafy vegetables, cereal grains, meats, cheeses, eggs, soybeans, blueberries, figs and vegetable oils. You should be able to receive all the vitamin K you require by eating a balanced and varied diet.

The NIH in the USA suggests:

- An adult male requires 120mcg of vitamin K daily
- An adult female requires 90mcg of vitamin K daily

The NHS in the UK suggests:

- An adult requires 1mcg of vitamin K for each kilogram of body weight, daily. Therefore, a person weighing 60kg would require 60mcg of vitamin K daily.

## *Mineral – Calcium*

Calcium is a mineral the body requires to keep bones strong and healthy, as well as for a number of other functions. These include muscle movement and for nerves to be able to carry messages from the brain to all parts of the body. Virtually all calcium is retained and stored in our bones and teeth, where it assists their structure and firmness.

Calcium can be found in many food groups, and with a varied diet we should be able to receive all the calcium our bodies require. Calcium can be found in milk, cheese and other dairy foods, green leafy vegetables, anything made with fortified flour, fish with soft bones you eat and foods with added calcium.

The NIH in the USA suggests:

- An adult (19-50) requires 1000mg of calcium daily
- An adult male (51-70) requires 1000mg of calcium daily
- An adult female (51-70) requires 1200mg of calcium daily

The NHS in the UK suggests:

- An adult (19-64) requires 700mg of calcium daily

## *Mineral – Iron*

Iron is an essential mineral and is used in our bodies to make red blood cells, which carry oxygen around your body. Iron is also used to make myoglobin, which is a protein that provides oxygen to muscles throughout your body, as well as maintaining healthy cells, hair, skin and nails.

We should be able to receive all the iron we need from our diets. Iron is found in many different foods; these include red meats, beef liver, dried apricots, nuts, green leafy vegetables, fortified breakfast cereals, edamame beans, chickpeas, dark chocolate and raisins. Should you require an iron supplement, taking iron with vitamin C helps the body absorb the mineral, and taking wholefood iron is softer on the stomach.

Should the body have a lack of iron it can lead to serious health issues such as anaemia. Subsequently, too much iron in our systems can lead to organ damage. It is therefore important that you are aware of what you are consuming and that you are not going to extremes with the iron levels.

The NIH in the USA suggests:

- An adult male (19-50) requires 8mg of iron daily
- An adult female (19-50) requires 18mg of iron daily
- An adult (50+) requires 8mg of iron daily

The NHS in the UK suggests:

- An adult male (19+) requires 8.7mg of iron daily
- An adult female (19-50) requires 14.8mg of iron daily
- An adult female (50+) requires 8.7mg of iron daily

### Mineral – Magnesium

Magnesium is a mineral and is one of the most important micronutrients. Magnesium assists the body in turning the food we eat into energy, making protein, DNA and bone, and helps to regulate muscle and nerve function, blood sugar levels and blood pressure. This mineral certainly packs a punch!

Magnesium is found in a wide variety of foods that include: nuts, wholemeal bread, green leafy vegetables, dark chocolate, brown rice, bananas, fortified breakfast cereals, milk, yogurts and seeds. While magnesium is found in a number of foods, it is likely that you could still be below the RDA. It is also available as a supplement and can be found in most multivitamin-mineral supplements.

The NIH in the USA suggests:

- An adult male (19+) requires 400-420mg of magnesium daily
- An adult female requires 310-320mg of magnesium daily

The NHS in the UK suggests:

- An adult male (19-64) requires 300mg of magnesium daily
- An adult female (19-64) requires 270mg of magnesium daily

## *Mineral – Zinc*

Zinc is an essential trace mineral that the body and immune system need daily to be healthy. Essential trace elements only require a small amount to be consumed for the body to receive its full health benefits.

Zinc is a powerful nutrient that is found in cells throughout the body and is crucial to the immune system in defending itself from bacteria and viruses. Zinc is also used in the body to make DNA and proteins, help wounds to heal, reduce inflammation and process carbohydrates, fats and proteins in food.

Zinc can be found in many food groups and with a varied diet we should be able to receive all the zinc our bodies require. It is found in red meats, shellfish, poultry, fish, dairy foods, breads, wheatgerm, nuts, seeds, beans and root vegetables. As the body does not store excess zinc, it must be consumed regularly as part of a healthy immune-friendly diet. It is also available as a supplement and can be found in most multivitamin-mineral supplements.

The NIH in the USA suggests:

- An adult male (19+) requires 11mg of zinc daily
- An adult female (19+) requires 8mg of zinc daily

The NHS in the UK suggests:

- An adult male (19-64) requires 9.5mg of zinc daily
- An adult female (19-64) requires 7mg of zinc daily

### *Warning! Seek Professional Guidance*

It is recommended to consult with a qualified naturopath or nutritionist before self-supplementing, especially if you suffer with a pre-existing health condition, as they will be able to advise you on the most appropriate dose for your needs. Those with chronic kidney disease or who are pregnant should not take supplements unless prescribed by their doctor.

# Simple Steps To Improve Your Immune System – Herbs

Our bodies can receive nutrients and immune boosters from a number of natural elements, including herbs, roots, plants and more. Throughout this chapter we take a closer look at some of the most well-known, researched and effective immune boosters that are readily available.

## *Echinacea*

Echinacea or coneflower is a pink or purple flower with nine known species, all of which are native to North America.

Echinacea is commonly taken as a means to protect the body, or defend it, from the common cold and similar infections. It is suggested that echinacea stimulates the immune system into increasing the white blood count in our body, which in turn fights infections more effectively and efficiently.

Echinacea should be taken when you believe you may be coming down with a cold or the flu. While short-term use of echinacea can offer some defence against the common cold, echinacea is not recommended to be used over a long period of time. This guidance has been given by the National Center for Complementary and Integrative Health (NCCIH), and by the World Health Organization, as it can have negative health effects.

## *Elderberry*

Elderberry is a dark purple berry that comes from the European or black elder tree. These trees are native to warmer climates in Europe, North America, Asia and northern Africa.

Elderberry has been used for many years as a form of

medicine and preliminary research from the NIH suggests that Elderberry may relieve symptoms of flu, colds and other upper-respiratory infections. It has been suggested that Elderberry could have a positive effect on COVID-19, although evidence is thus far limited.

The dark purple Elderberry is packed with antioxidants, vitamins and antiviral compounds that boost your immune system. It has also been said to reduce inflammation in the body. While supplements are available, teas and syrups made from the Elderberry plant/berry are often used.

## Panax Ginseng

Panax ginseng comes from the root area of several plants in the Panax family. There are two types of ginseng: Asian ginseng called Panax Ginseng and American ginseng called Panax Quinquefolius. Research on both plants has found that the American ginseng is not as potent as its Asian cousin.

Panax ginseng contains two significant elements (ginsenosides and gintonin) that come together to provide excellent health benefits. As a powerful antioxidant, Panax ginseng has been found to be an effective healer in reducing inflammation throughout the body. It has also been found to boost the immune system (fighting colds), improve brain function and focus, regulate blood sugar and improve erectile dysfunction.

Panax ginseng is taken as a supplement as there are no natural food sources of ginseng. These are usually taken as a tea, a powder, capsules or dried herbs. It is possible to find some energy foods and drinks with added Panax ginseng.

## Propolis

Propolis, along with honey and royal jelly, is made by bees. It is made of resin (50%), wax (30%), essential oils (10%), pollen (5%)

and other organic compounds (5%). Propolis is often known as 'bee-glue' and is used to seal holes and cracks, and for the restoration of beehives.

A study led by Visweswara Rao Passupuleti from the Institute of Food Security and Sustainable Agriculture (Malaysia) found that Propolis had many biological efficacies including anti-cancer, antibacterial, antifungal, antioxidant, antidiabetic, anti-inflammatory and dental action. This is one powerful immune-boosting herb!

Propolis is used for a multitude of ills. It is a great natural product for mouth sores, ulcers and any inflammation. It can assist with abdominal pain, diarrhoea, bloating and nausea. It is used in many creams and gels, as a wound healing agent for acne, cuts, burns and sores of all types. Not least, it is a great boost to the immune system, especially in times of colds, flu, sore throats and sinus pain.

## Sage

Sage comes from the sage plant and is a herb used throughout cooking, as well as for its health benefits. Sage comes from the mint family and has a sweet and savoury flavour. It has been used as a herbal remedy since the era of the ancient Greeks and Romans.

Sage has a number of antibacterial, antioxidant and anti-inflammatory properties, meaning it has been effective in easing congestions from chest infections, coughs and respiratory issues. It is also regularly used to reduce a sore mouth and throat, increase memory and brain function, lower cholesterol and reduce blood sugar levels.

Sage can be used in a number of varieties, including fresh or dried. It is often used in homemade remedies and teas, and can also be included in your diet as a garnish or seasoning for roasts, meats and stews.

## *Thyme*

Thyme is a similar herb to Sage; it is part of the mint family and is well known for the pungent aroma of its dried leaves and flowering tops. It is also used in the culinary world as well as for its health benefits.

Thyme has incredible antibacterial, insecticidal and antimicrobial properties. That means it is an effective herb in treating inflammation, bacterial and fungal infections, patchy hair loss, stomach issues, and reducing blood pressure and respiratory infections, such as bronchitis.

Thyme can be consumed in foods, and is present in oils, perfumes, soaps, cosmetics and toothpastes. For health benefits, Thyme is best consumed in a thyme tea, using fresh thyme leaves, or in cooking.

## *Turmeric*

Turmeric comes from the ginger family and is native to southeast Asia. It has been used in Indian medicines and cooking for thousands of years and has tremendous health benefits.

Turmeric was also used across Eastern Asian medicine, including Chinese. Within these medical systems, turmeric was used for skin disorders, wound healing, joint problems (arthritis etc.), to reduce inflammation, upper respiratory issues and stomach/digestive disorders.

While turmeric has been used for centuries, modern research suggests that turmeric has positive antibacterial, anti-inflammatory, anti-cancer and antioxidant effects on the body. It is therefore often recommended for liver disease, arthritis, cancers, respiratory infections, wound healing, diabetes, depression, allergies, to boost the immune system and more.

Turmeric is not often found in everyday foods in the Western hemisphere; however, dietary supplements, drinks and foods are available. Turmeric has been found to be poorly absorbed by the body. It is therefore recommended to find a supplement that includes black pepper as this increases the absorption rate.

## Wild Cherry Bark

Wild cherry bark comes from the black cherry tree, which is native to eastern and central North America. It has been used for many hundreds of years, including by the Native Americans. It was originally used to relieve coughs, diarrhoea, labour pains and respiratory issues. It was also used as a general sedative.

Wild cherry bark is often found as a key ingredient in cough syrups and other remedies for respiratory conditions. The bark acts as an expectorant, helping to expel mucus from the lungs and to dry excess moisture. It is packed with zinc, iron, potassium and calcium. As wild cherry bark has antiviral, antitussive, antibacterial and anti-cancer properties, it is often used for many illnesses that affect the respiratory or digestive systems.

Wild cherry bark is not something that is found in our diets naturally and therefore needs to be introduced additionally. It is best used in a hot tea blend, tincture or syrup. The fresher the wild cherry bark the better, as it will pack a more potent and effective punch.

## Warning! Seek Professional Guidance

It is recommended that you consult with a qualified herbalist, naturopath or nutritionist before self-supplementing, especially if you suffer with a pre-existing health condition, as they will be able to advise you on the most appropriate dose for your needs. Those with chronic kidney disease or who are pregnant should not take supplements unless prescribed by their doctor.

# Steps Together

## Specialist Drug And Alcohol Rehabilitation Group

This chapter has been edited with the assistance of Steps Together. Steps Together is a private specialist drug and alcohol rehabilitation group with centres set in tranquil environments.

As part of Steps Together's drug or alcohol detox programme, their chef prepares high quality healthy meals in keeping with their programme, and ensures each person 'feels' healthy and relaxed.

If you are in need of advice, contact Steps Together for a confidential conversation.

Use this reference when making contact:
THE HOLISTIC GUIDE

Website: https://stepstogether.rehab
UK Phone: 0800 038 5585
Email: info@stepstogether.rehab

# Mind Over Matter:
# A Matter Of The Mind

*Mental health problems don't define who you are. They are something you experience. You walk in the rain and you feel the rain, but, importantly, YOU ARE NOT THE RAIN.*
Matt Haig

# Mental Health And The Immune System

In 2020, the World Health Organization, United for Global Mental Health and the World Federation for Mental Health made a joint statement in which they stated that mental health is one of the most neglected areas of public health, with close to one billion people currently living with a mental health disorder. It is estimated that over 3 million people die every year from the harmful use of alcohol, and one person dies every 40 seconds by suicide. Despite this, many countries spend, on average, only 2% of their health budgets on mental health.

Our human bodies have many differing systems (physical, mental, energetic and emotional) that keep us running and working well, most of these have been heavily researched. What is still fairly unknown are the relationships between the health systems. There is continuing evidence that our bodies work in complete harmony, and any disease in any system can manifest into either a physical, mental, energetic or emotional disease.

## The History Of The Mind-Body Connection

The connection between the mind and body has been known in some form for many centuries, dating back to the second century with physicians Galen and Moses Maimonides. Both understood that emotions affect physical health. While the connection between the mind and body has been known, it has only been researched in more depth over the past 40 years, and we still have some way to go yet.

While it has been evidenced that the Eastern world has long understood and focused on the energies of our bodies, the Western medical world has been slower to embrace the positive effects of mindfulness and the energetic system. It was the well-known Canadian physician, one of the three founders of the Johns Hopkins Medical School, Sir William Osler (1849-1919), who first penned in his textbook *Principles and Practice of Medicine* that our minds can be tricked or duped into having genuine physical responses and reactions to artificial elements. In his research, Sir William wrote about a patient who had an asthma attack from smelling an artificial rose. He found that an asthma attack could be induced by either direct nervous system stimulation or via psychological nervous system stimulation. This was the first known medical example of the mind-body connection. These findings led us to further studies and have resulted in understanding much of what we know today.

It was in 1975 that Sir William Osler's findings were scientifically explained by Dr Robert Ader of the University of Rochester. Through scientific studies, Dr Ader was aiming to understand Sir William's research of how our minds can be fooled into having a physical reaction or response to a non-genuine object.

Dr Ader's results were outstanding, ground-breaking even. He was able to provide the first scientific proof that our emotions and thoughts alter the way in which our immune system works and reacts. This was the first piece of evidence that proved that our bodily systems interact with each other. Until this moment in history, it was thought that our bodily systems worked independently of each other.

In today's modern world, it is now completely understandable, and rational, to believe that each of our bodily systems, while having their own functions, work in unison with each other to create our total health. What therefore becomes comprehensive is that as a human being, we must take complete care of our wellbeing, which means looking after our physical, mental, energetic and emotional health.

## The Modern Mind-Body Connection

A publication from 2006 by Vicki Brower on mind-body research highlights research that helps close the gap on the link between health and emotions, behaviours, social and economic status and personality. In the publication, Oakley Ray, Professor Emeritus of Psychology, Psychiatry and Pharmacology at Vanderbilt University, states that:

*According to the mind-body or biopsychosocial paradigm, which supersedes the older biomedical model, there is no real division between mind and body because of networks of communication that exist between the brain and neurological, endocrine and immune systems.*

In short, the connection between our mind and body is interlinked by the networks that keep us alive and healthy. Without one, the other cannot work effectively and efficiently.

Further studies have been conducted and found an evidence-based link between physical health and mental stress. Research conducted by Jill Littrell PhD, School of Social Work, Georgia State University, states that stress alters white blood cell function. When stressed, the response of white blood cells to viral infected cells and cancer cells decreases. Additionally, when we are stressed, wound healing is impacted and any vaccinations received during this time are less effective.

In the early 1980s, Dr Dean Ornish, Clinical Professor of Medicine at the University of California, claimed that heart disease could be prevented and potentially reversed with 'lifestyle changes', which included a mixture of a very low-fat vegetarian diet, meditation/yoga, moderate exercise, stress management and social support. While he was treated with some contempt by his peers at the time, his theory was later proven to have merit, sparking further studies of the effects of the mind-body connection. Studies by David Spiegel (1980), Nemeroff et al (1998), Goodwin et al (2001), Kissane et al (2004), Sunquist et al (2005), Antoni et al (2006) and Carlson et al (2014) found considerable evidence of improvement from headaches, chronic lower-back pain, incontinence, cancer symptoms (and recovery) and coronary artery disease when using mind-body treatments.

One final example of mind over matter is the placebo effect. A placebo is something that seems to be a genuine medical treatment; however, it is usually a harmless replacement. Professor Ted Kaptchuk, of the Harvard-affiliated Beth Israel Deaconess Medical Center, believes that:

*The placebo effect is more than positive thinking – believing a treatment or procedure will work. It's about creating a stronger connection between the brain and body and how they work together.*

Our mind can have a powerful effect on our physical body.

Dr James Gordon, a Harvard-educated psychiatrist and founder of the Center for Mind-Body Medicine, concludes that the mind-body connection is more than the connective combination of the physical and mental bodies. Dr Gordon suggests that:

*The brain and peripheral nervous system, the endocrine and immune systems, and indeed, all the organs of our body and all the emotional responses we have, share a common chemical language and are constantly communicating with one another.*

Our physical, mental, energetic and emotional health are intertwined in what is known as the mind-body connection.

## What Is Mental Health?

We all have mental health, in the same way as we all have physical health. Whereas physical health refers to our bodies, mental health focuses on our behavioural, emotional and cognitive wellbeing.

According to the World Health Organization,

*Mental Health is a state of wellbeing in which an individual realises his or her own abilities, can cope with the normal stresses of life, can work productively, and is able to make a contribution to his or her community.*

It is as important to take care of the wellbeing and health of our minds as it is the wellbeing and health of our body. In short, mental health is our current state of mind, and the ability to cope with life's stresses and challenges. It is very likely that everyone will go through low or difficult mental moments in life; however, it is continuous episodes of mental ill health, finding it difficult to manage how to think, feel or react to daily stresses, that could be a sign of poor mental health and an indication of a wider problem.

Should you have signs of poor mental health, it does not mean you or someone else is mentally ill, this is something quite different. Mental health affects everyone and requires daily self-management. Having good mental health means more than not having issues surrounding you, it is part of the holistic health of you.

According to the 2013 Global Burden of Disease study, the predominant mental health issue worldwide is depression, followed by anxiety, schizophrenia and bipolar disorder. The study also found that depression was the second leading cause of years lived with disability worldwide, behind lower-back pain, and that depression was the primary driver of disability in 26 countries worldwide.

## Are Mental Health Issues Common?

According to the World Health Organization, one in four people will experience or be affected by ill mental health at some point in their lives. Mental health problems are common throughout society and are the reason why every person needs to continuously manage their mental health.

In our lives we can face challenging moments that include bereavement, divorce, financial issues, losing a job, social problems...these moments are often short-lived, although they can have a lasting impact on our mental health. With the support of friends, family and professionals (if needed), we are able to take the necessary steps to make a positive recovery.

While mental health issues are said to affect 25% of the world's population, a smaller percentage of the population will be affected by more serious mental health issues.

Serious mental health problems can be linked to a history of mental illness in the family bloodline and are often triggered by specific events or moments in a person's life. These events can lead to changes in a person's behaviour, thoughts or beliefs, as well as eating and drinking habits.

# What Constitutes A Mental Health Disorder?

There are a number of different mental health disorders that are recognised as an official illness or disease by the likes of the National Institutes of Health (US), Public Health England (UK) and other governmental health organisations globally. I have listed a number of these disorders below for your reference and further personal research.

- Addiction disorders – alcohol, drugs, gambling, sex, shopping
- Attention deficit hyperactivity disorder (ADHD)
- Anxiety disorders
- Bipolar disorder
- Conduct disorders – kleptomania, pyromania
- Depression – a cause for disease or a reaction to disease
- Eating disorders – clinical anorexia and bulimia
- Fear – suppresses the immune system
- Gender dysphoria
- Insomnia
- Munchausen's syndrome
- Neurocognitive disorders – Alzheimer's, traumatic brain injury
- Obsessive-Compulsive Disorder (OCD)
- Personality disorders
- Pervasive developmental disorders
- Phobias – agoraphobia, social, arachnophobia etc.
- Postnatal depression
- Post-traumatic stress disorder (PTSD)
- Psychosis
- Schizoaffective disorder
- Schizophrenia
- Seasonal affective disorder (SAD)
- Stress – one of the world's biggest killers

## Who Does Mental Health Affect?

In a global health study from 2017 by the Institute for Health Metrics and Evaluation – and reported in their flagship Global Burden of Disease study – they estimated that over 792 million people lived with a mental disorder, which is just over 10% of the global population. That is, one in ten people on the planet lives with some form of mental illness. They estimate that:

- Anxiety disorders account for 284 million cases globally
- Depression accounts for 264 million cases globally
- Bipolar disorders account for 46 million cases globally
- Schizophrenia accounts for 20 million cases globally
- Eating disorders (clinical anorexia and bulimia) account for 16 million cases globally

The Global Burden of Disease study also estimates that alongside mental health, the number of people globally who have a substance use disorder equates to 178 million people.

- Alcohol use accounts for 107 million cases globally
- Drug use accounts for 71 million cases globally

Addiction is described as a compulsive and repetitive disorder that is characterised by repeated use of drugs, or the repetitive engagement in activities such as gambling, sex, alcohol, social media, food, Internet, video games…regardless of the negative effects to self and harm to others. Public Health England see addiction as a disease.

When you combine the number of mental health sufferers with those with an addiction disorder, it takes the total number of people globally who suffer from any mental or substance use disorder to a staggering 970 million people, 13% of the global population (12.6% of males and 13.3% of females). It is possible that the number is far greater than this, especially when you consider the effects of COVID-19 and the lockdowns of 2020/21.

## How Mental Health Affects Physical Health

Through medical research conducted, we have been able to understand in more detail how the impact on our mental health has an effect on our physical health.

An independent charitable organisation working to improve health and care in England, called The King's Fund, suggests that mental health problems significantly increase the risk of poor physical health, just as poor physical health can significantly increase the risk of poor mental health.

A study produced by King's College London analysed data from 3.2 million people living with severe mental illness. It found that those suffering with a severe mental illness were 53% more likely to be affected by a cardiovascular disease than those without a mental illness.

It has been found that those with extreme levels of stress and distress are 32% more likely to die from cancer, compared to those with minimal levels of distress.

Medical research has found that depression is linked to a 50% increase in the risk of a person dying from cancer and a 67% increase in the risk of a person dying from a type of heart disease. According to the NIH, scientists have discovered that people with depression show signs of increased inflammation in the body, changes in the control of heart rate and blood circulation, abnormalities in stress hormones and metabolic changes.

A 2014 study led by Petter Andreas Ringen on 'Increased Mortality in Schizophrenia Due to Cardiovascular Disease' concluded that schizophrenia sufferers are likely to have a reduced lifespan of 15 to 20 years. There are links that show that Schizophrenia can increase the risk of death from heart disease by 40-50%, and increase the risk of death from respiratory disease by 66%.

## What Are Some Factors That Can Affect Mental Health?

Our mental health and our ability to cope with life's stresses differs from person to person. Whereas some people never seem to get fazed by what is thrown at them, others can be more affected by life situations.

There are a number of potential causes of mental health issues. It is often a combination of factors that come together to act as a major catalyst for an individual's mental health to be affected.

The following have been highlighted as the most common factors that can affect our mental health:

- Being a long-term carer for someone
- Bereavement (losing someone close to you)
- Childhood abuse, trauma or neglect
- Coming from a one-parent family
- Domestic violence, bullying or other abuse as an adult
- Experiencing discrimination and stigma
- Having a long-term physical health condition
- History of mental health in the family bloodline (genetics)
- Homelessness or poor housing
- Life experiences (COVID-19)
- Sleeping problems
- Serious physical injury (head or brain injury)
- Severe or long-term stress
- Smoking, drug, gambling and alcohol misuse
- Social disadvantage, poverty or debt
- Social isolation or loneliness
- Trauma as an adult (military combat, threat to life)
- Losing your job or business

While it is possible that lifestyle factors can have an effect on our mental health, it is likely that experiencing a mental health issue will usually stem from other areas as well.

## COVID-19 And Its Effect On Mental Health

To say that 2020 was a challenging year is something of an understatement. No matter who you are or where you live, everyone has been affected to some degree by COVID-19 and the global pandemic that engulfed us all. A study conducted by Oracle and Workplace Intelligence in 2020 questioned more than 12,000 working professionals across 11 countries to assess mental stresses, anxieties and burnouts throughout the COVID-19 pandemic.

The results from the study show a small sample of the mental impact that COVID-19 and lockdowns have had on the human population, including fear, worry and anxiety.

### *COVID-19 And The Impact On The Global Workforce*

- 70% of people had more stress and anxiety at work in 2020
- 78% said their mental health was negatively impacted
- 38% said they had a lack of work-life balance
- 25% felt burnt out (overworked)
- 25% felt depressed from lack of socialisation
- 14% suffered with loneliness
- 42% struggled with pressures of performance standards
- 41% struggled with handling routine and tedious tasks
- 41% struggled to juggle unmanageable workloads

### *COVID-19 And The Impact On Home Life*

- 85% of people said that mental health issues affect home life
- 40% said that they were sleep deprived
- 35% said that they had poor physical health
- 33% were less happy at home

- 30% said that family relationships were suffering
- 28% felt isolated from friends
- 62% said that they prefer remote home working
- 51% have more time to spend with their family
- 30% said they could get more work done

## Stress And The Immune System

Stress is widely known to have a negative effect on the body. Dr Sheldon Cohen PhD et al, at the Department of Psychology, Carnegie Mellon University, Pittsburgh, conducted a study in 1991 that concluded that stress suppresses a person's defences against infection and increases the infection's rate of growth, which makes us more susceptible to colds, flu and other viruses. A further study by Ronald Glaser and Janice Kiecolt-Glaser (2005) also concluded that stressful life events can dysregulate the immune response.

Being chronically stressed, especially over a long period of time, can result in us developing autoimmune and inflammatory disorders. When we are stressed, our bodies produce additional amounts of the hormone cortisol. Cortisol produced in larger quantities can negatively affect how the body regulates its inflammatory response, which can lead to it attacking its own immune system, causing the development of autoimmune, inflammatory disorders and other negative effects.

In 2019, Annina Seiler, Christopher P. Fagundes and Lisa M. Christian published 'The Impact of Everyday Stressors on the Immune System and Health'. They concluded that chronic stress has a number of ill effects on the body. When chronically stressed our bodies' defences are lowered, making us more susceptible to infectious illnesses, poor wound healing, a slower immune response to viruses, a weaker response to vaccines and an increase in inflammatory processes.

When the body is affected in this way it can increase the risk of a number of physical and mental disorders; these include diabetes, autoimmune disease, cardiovascular disease, inflammatory disorders, frailty and a reduced lifespan. These findings by Seiler, Fagundes and Christian provide evidence to suggest that chronic stress and immune dysregulation can contribute to serious adverse health issues.

## Managing Stress Boosts Your Immune System

Managing stress is not only about going for a long walk through nature, or meditating regularly. It is about understanding and knowing yourself, mentally, physically and emotionally. The more you understand the whole of you, the better you will be able to manage all aspects of life. Continuously managing stress levels, regardless of how much or little you experience, can help your immune system fight off germs and viruses.

The study of 'Psychoneuroimmunology: Psychological Influences on Immune Function and Health' by psychologist Janice Kiecolt-Glaser PhD and immunologist Ronald Glaser PhD compared the immune functions of medical students undertaking stressful medical exams who had been given hypnosis and relaxation training, with those students undertaking the same exams without the hypnosis and relaxation training.

The evidence of the study was conclusive. Those students who followed the hypnosis and relaxation training on a continuous basis were found to have a significantly stronger immune function throughout the exam period when compared to those students who either had no training or who trained inconsistently.

Spending time meditating, using deep breathing techniques, walking in nature, talking about personal issues, spending time with close friends are key to our overall health. It is vitally important that every person makes time for themselves and spends time with themselves. These moments, and connection to self, are invaluable for your mental, physical, energetic and emotional health.

# What Are Some Of The Signs Of Poor Mental Health?

Should you recognise a number of these signs in yourself, a friend, colleague or family member, it is important to seek advice and support.

- Being anxious, irritable and short-tempered
- Being overly suspicious and paranoid
- Being easily distracted
- Being overly aggressive
- Being overwhelmed by things and situations
- Being isolated and withdrawn
- Being less talkative
- Believing your family and friends want to do you harm
- Believing that people or organisations are out to get you
- Believing in wild conspiracy theories
- Believing that you have special powers or are on a mission
- Excessive spending and problems managing your money
- Excessive eating
- Feeling overly frustrated
- Feeling the need to drink more alcohol
- Feeling overly emotional, sad and/or teary
- Feeling continuously low
- Feeling like you have a lack of energy
- Finding it difficult to concentrate
- Finding it difficult to make decisions
- Having difficulty sleeping
- Having difficulty getting out of bed
- Having difficulty with memory loss
- Having mood swings
- Having suicidal thoughts
- Having hallucinations

- Speaking erratically with no consistent thought
- Struggling with daily chores
- Struggling to manage your emotions
- Worrying excessively

# What Treatments And Support Are Available?

There are a number of treatments that are available to those with mental health issues; these include prescribed medications, energy therapies, light therapies and psychological therapies. I have listed a number of these treatments below for your reference and further personal research.

## *Prescribed Medications And Treatments*

- Antianxiety medications
- Antidepressants
- Antipsychotics
- Electroconvulsive therapy
- Mood stabilisers
- Tranquilisers
- Transcranial magnetic stimulation
- Treatment in a hospital or clinic
- Vagus nerve stimulation

## *Psychological Therapies*

- Art therapy
- Autogenic training
- Behavioural therapy
- Biofeedback
- Cognitive behavioural therapy
- Community self-help groups (Anonymous meetings)
- Counselling and couples therapy
- Dance
- Deep breathing techniques
- Dialectical behaviour therapy
- Eye movement desensitisation and retrocession
- Family therapy

- Group therapy
- HeartMath therapy
- Humour/laughter
- Hypnotherapy
- Hypnagogia
- Imagery
- Individual therapy
- Interpersonal therapy
- Love and affection
- Meditation or yoga
- Neurolinguistic programming
- Psychoanalysis
- Psychodynamic psychotherapy
- Supportive psychotherapy
- Writing therapy

## *Energy Therapies*

- Acupuncture
- Applied kinesiology
- Curanderos and curanderas
- Healing traditions of indigenous peoples
- Homeopathy
- Kahuna
- Polarity therapy
- Prayer and spiritual healing
- Qigong
- Reiki
- Therapeutic touch
- Thought field therapy

## *Light And Rhythm Therapies*

- Auriculotherapy

- Bioacoustics
- Colour therapy
- Full-spectrum and bright-light therapy
- Laser acupuncture
- Medical resonance therapy music
- Music entertainment and music therapy
- Tomatis
- Ultraviolet therapy

# Steps Together

## Specialist Drug And Alcohol Rehabilitation Group

This chapter has been edited with the assistance of Steps Together. Steps Together is a private specialist drug and alcohol rehabilitation group with centres set in tranquil environments.

Steps Together's team consists of some of the UK's most experienced and qualified counsellors and practitioners in drug and alcohol addiction treatment. Their philosophy is to help you, or a loved one, become sober and drug free. Helping to build a life of hope and freedom for the future.

If you are in need of advice, contact Steps Together for a confidential conversation.

Use this reference when making contact:
**THE HOLISTIC GUIDE**

Website: https://stepstogether.rehab
UK Phone: 0800 038 5585
Email: info@stepstogether.rehab

# Feeling The Flow Of The Energy Within

*Comprehensive healthcare must involve thorough attention to the mind and spirit, not only the body.*
Leonard Wisneski and Lucy Anderson

# The Energetic System And The Immune System

## Introduction – The Energetic System And The 7 Chakras

This chapter has been edited with the assistance of Sara Leslie, International Spiritual Clairvoyant, Medium and Healer. You can find further information on Sara Leslie at the end of the chapter.

Our bodies are an integrated system that combines the physical, mental, emotional and energetic body, working together as one.

There are differing scholastic views of the true origins of the chakra system. In the West, it is agreed by most that the chakra system dates back to India between the 1500s and 500s BCE and comes from the Hindu-Brahmin oral tradition of Vedas (considered to be the oldest written texts of Hinduism). The first written account of chakra/s were found in the Vedas. There are many Indian scholars who believe that the chakra system is far older than the 1500s BCE, and that the original masters and teachers passed this knowledge down to their students through an oral tradition long before Indo-Europeans journeyed to India.

Within Eastern spiritual traditions, where the study of chakras originated, it is believed that the seven primary chakras are the basis of our human existence. The Western approach to the 7 chakras emphasises each chakra as a different aspect of life in the modern world, often describing their function in terms comprising of the physical, psychological, energetic and spiritual.

The word Chakra is pronounced sharr-kra.

## What Is A Chakra?

The Vedas, where the first written account of chakras was found, are written entirely in Sanskrit words. The direct translation of Chakra from Sanskrit means wheel, disc, vortex or turning. Chakra is believed to have been associated with the chariot wheels of the ruler Cakravartin, who in Sanskrit is referred to as an ideal universal king who rules ethically and benevolently over the entire world.

Chakras are said to be wheels or discs of energy that permeate from seven specific points on the physical body. The chakras are constantly rotating as energy passes through us in a figure-of-8 that repeats on itself. These seven points on the body are the main areas for the reception, connection and transmission of energies. It is believed by Hinduism practitioners and those of New Age Spirituality that chakras interact with the ductless endocrine gland and lymphatic system in the physical body. By interacting together, it is said that chakras feed in good bio-energies and dispose of unwanted bio-energies.

For a number of people, the idea of chakras or an energetic system can seem far-fetched. Anything other than what can been seen, touched or heard can be hard to believe at times. Seeing, after all, is believing. Isn't it?

The short answer is no. We are electrical beings. Electricity, and therefore energy, plays a vital part in our ability to live and function. For example, the heart is the strongest electrical generator in the body, where the flow of charged ions causes your heart to beat and your muscles to contract. Similarly, the brain is a constant hotbed of electrical activity that contains in the region of a hundred billion electrically conductive biological wires. If you are still not convinced, in many medical fields our electrical frequencies and impulses, including ESG and MRI, are measured to assess our physical health.

## The Chakra Systems

There are various chakras systems, depending on your beliefs and understanding. These systems range from the most commonly known 7 chakra system, to a 9, 12, 13, 16 and 22 chakra system. It is widely acknowledged that the chakras 1-7 relate to the physical body, whereas 8 to 22 focus on the energetic and spiritual.

According to Dr Amit Ray PhD, the author of several books on meditation, there are 114 chakras and 72,000 Nadis in the human body. He describes Nadis as pathways of life energies and chakras as the purification and distribution centres of life energies in our body. Chakras and Nadis are said to be highly connected with the four forms of energies in life – physical, mental, emotional and spiritual energy. Dr Ray believes for a healthy and 'perfect' life we need complete balance of all four energies, with chakras playing an important role in balancing these energies.

The 7 chakra system is the most widely used in the Western world and is made of seven energy focal points or centres. These energy centres are located along the spine, starting at the base of the spine through to the top of the head. As said above, chakras 1-7 are connected to the physical body and are each individually connected to specific physical elements, including endocrine glands, organs and nerve areas.

In every chakra system each chakra has its own individuality and will have differing energetic, emotional and physical effects. Every chakra has its own colour and vibrational frequency, as well as its own connection to Elements (earth, wind, water, fire and space), Gemstones (Ruby, Sapphire, Emerald, etc.) and Stars (Sun, Moon, Jupiter, etc.).

## The 7 Chakra System

Using the diagram below, we can see where each of the 7 chakras are located throughout the body, along the spine. Additionally, each of chakras are named individually below.

1st Chakra – Muladhara – Root
2nd Chakra – Svadhishthana – Sacral
3rd Chakra – Manipura – Solar Plexus
4th Chakra – Anahata – Heart
5th Chakra – Vishuddha – Throat
6th Chakra – Ajna – Third Eye
7th Chakra – Sahasrara – Crown

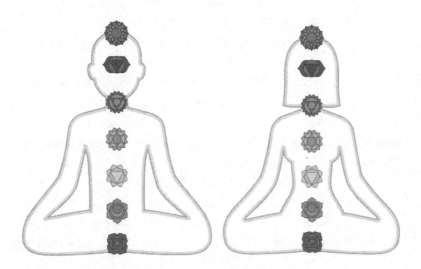

## The Connection Between Mind, Body And Energy

Many years of research have been spent on understanding the connection between our minds and our physical bodies, and the effects thereof. The book *The Scientific Basis of Integrative Medicine* by Leonard Wisneski MD and Lucy Anderson states that the connection between mind and body is so entwined that,

> *comprehensive healthcare must involve thorough attention to the mind and spirit, not only the body. In order for Western medicine to have a cohesive physiological system, it must account for the existence of energy fields within as well as outside of the human body.*

It is clear that we must spend as much time focusing on our minds, and energy fields, as we do on our bodies.

Wisneski and Anderson present evidence to suggest that the pineal gland is the link between the internal body systems and our external environment. They believe that the pineal gland takes outside environmental information and translates it into chemical and electrical signals throughout our bodily systems.

The pineal gland is often called the third eye and is considered to be mysterious, with links to spirit and the sixth sense. Human knowledge of the pineal gland has been dated as far back as Ancient Egypt (Tutankhamun). Many artefacts have been found throughout this time period with the pineal gland evident; these include statues, necklaces and hieroglyphics.

Over the past 30 years or so the pineal gland, and its function, has been better understood by scientists. Studies reveal that the functions of the pineal gland include: the secretion of melatonin, converting temperature, light and magnetic environmental information into neuroendocrine signals that regulate and control functions within the body, and regulating our internal body clock, which assists in our daily sleep and wake patterns, as well as with daily routines in our busy lives.

Our physical, mental and energetic body works as one.

## How Do Chakras Work?

Chakras are often described as wheels of energy, and they have an important task in the complete system of our health. Chakras are the entrance point and pathways for which subtle energy can be introduced into the body and then transferred into an energy form that can be used at a cellular level.

Dr Amit Ray PhD says that chakras have seven states that are actively changing due to the chakra's interaction with the external and internal environment. The seven states of the chakra are: open, closed, excessive open, balanced, active, underactive and overactive.

In the book *The Scientific Basis of Integrative Medicine* by Leonard Wisneski MD and Lucy Anderson, the authors have evidenced that the subtle energy received by the chakras is transferred into hormones and neurotransmitters for the body to use. The chakras are able to control the energy flows throughout the electrical network in our physical body and have a similarity to how the pineal gland interacts with the body.

As we have understood previously, the pineal gland converts light, temperature and magnetic environmental information for our body to use. In effect, the pineal gland is the energy transducer for our bodily senses, sending hormonal and electrical messages throughout the body. In a similar manner, the chakras are the energy transducers for subtle energy. In the 7 chakra system, each of the 7 chakras are a receptor for subtle energy; that energy is converted into other forms of energy and directed throughout the body. Each chakra correlates to physical bodily systems (endocrine glands and major nerve areas) and plays an important role in our complete health by regulating the complicated system of energy that passes through the body.

In Chinese medicine, the energy that passes through our body is referred to as Qi, which when translated into English means *life force* or *vital energy*. The chakras are constantly rotating as energy passes through us in a figure-8 that repeats on itself, connecting into the autonomic nervous system where it then interacts magnificently with the endocrine system. The seventh chakra is connected differently to the other six chakras. The seventh chakra is located at the top or crown of the head and is connected with the pineal gland and central nervous system. It is understood that the seventh chakra connects via the central nervous system to the autonomic nervous system and then to the endocrine system.

In 1977, two scientific researchers, Roger Guillemin and Andrew V. Schally, discovered the first hypothalamic secretion of hormones. This finding was ground-breaking. Until Guillemin and Schally made their discovery scientists had not considered the brain as an endocrine organ. Due to their findings, scientists have continued to discover new hormones and neurotransmitters. Guillemin and Schally both won the Nobel Prize for their research.

The endocrine system is a network of glands that stretches throughout the body and is in control of producing, regulating and distributing hormones to regulate the metabolism and a number of other bodily functions. The endocrine system turns an electrical signal into the evolution of a single or multiple hormones, which are then guided throughout various parts of the body, communicating and directing functional bodily activity. The endocrine system includes the following glands: parathyroid, thyroid, pancreas, adrenals, thymus, hypothalamus, pituitary, gonads (ovaries and testes) and the pineal gland.

These 7 points on the body are the main areas for the reception, connection and transmission of energies. The chakras that relate to each of the seven areas must remain clear for the energy to pass through us efficiently and to be used effectively by the body. It is possible for the chakras to become blocked by everyday stresses, emotional strains and physical issues. When blocked, the chakras are unable to regulate the energy flow in the body, causing an irregular and inconsistent energy flow which can lead to physical illness or mental/emotional imbalance.

According to Wisneski and Anderson, stress can be defined as,

> *the absence of homeostasis or an imbalance in the harmonious workings of the organism, which results in the body's concerted effort to re-establish that balance. The stress response triggers the release of powerful hormones that generate arousal and anxiety.*

In short, without control over everyday stressors it is likely that your chakras will become blocked, causing physical, mental and emotional irregularities.

What is clear from the abundance of research available to us, including that of Wisneski and Anderson, is that every human being needs a balance between the mind and the body, and a balanced flow of energy for complete health.

# The 7 Chakras

The individual chakras all have specific connections to the endocrine glands, major nerve areas and organs in our body, as well as a connection to colours, planets/stars and more. Below is a description of which chakra relates to which element. There is further detail on this within each chakra description.

## What Does It All Mean?

**Name:** this is the most widely recognised English name for the chakra

**Sanskrit Name:** the Sanskrit name for the chakra

**Sanskrit Translation:** this is the direct translation or closest English words to the translation

**Association:** the key focal point of the chakra

**Meaning:** this is the meaning and connection of the chakra to one's self

**Colour Vibration:** this is the colour of the vibration from the chakra's energy or the energy radiating from the chakra

**Element:** which earthly element is the chakra associated

**Planet/Star:** which planet/star is the chakra associated

**Gemstone:** which gemstone is the chakra associated. They emit positive energies & absorb negatives energies

**Bija Mantra:** when said aloud, this one-syllable sound activates the energy of the chakra to bring balance and healing power to the mind, body and soul

**Bija Mantra Sound:** how to pronounce the Bija Mantra

**Developmental Stage:** at what stage of life does this chakra's energy portal open

**Location:** what part of the body is the chakra located

**Cornerstone for Self:** the chakra's emotional connection to self

**Endocrine Glands:** the endocrine gland/s the chakra is connected to and physically affects

**Signs of Balance:** physical, mental and emotional signs that your chakra is in balance

**Physical Influences:** body organs the chakra is connected to and physically affects

**Physical Imbalance:** physical signs that your chakra is blocked

**Emotional Imbalance:** emotional signs that your chakra is blocked

**Unblocking Activities:** activities or actions you can take to unblock this chakra

**Cleansing Stones:** these gems have a vibrating energy that can clear or unblock your chakra (usually with a chakra energy clearing meditation)

## 1st Chakra – The Root Chakra

| | |
|---|---|
| **Name:** | Root Chakra |
| **Sanskrit name:** | Muladhara |
| **Sanskrit translation:** | Root or base |
| **Association:** | Birth, survival, safety and stability |
| **Meaning:** | I am |
| **Colour vibration:** | Red |
| **Element:** | Earth |
| **Planet/Star:** | Sun |
| **Gemstone:** | Ruby |
| **Bija mantra:** | LAM |
| **Bija mantra sound:** | L-U-U-U-M-M |
| **Developmental stage:** | Womb to 7 years old |
| **Location:** | At the base of the spine, on your tail bone, near the coccyx. |
| **Cornerstone for self:** | Stability, grounding, physical health, prosperity, honesty and trust. |
| **Endocrine glands:** | Adrenal glands and kidneys; regulates the immune system and metabolism. |
| **Physical influences:** | Coccyx (tail bone), lower back, hips, spine, legs, bones, feet, rectum, immune system, bone marrow, colon, kidneys and the adrenal glands. |
| **Signs of balance:** | You feel supported, a sense of connection and safety to the physical world, and you are well-grounded. You live a healthy lifestyle, with self-confidence and good physical energy. |
| **Physical imbalance:** | Having weight problems or eating disorders, knee, leg or feet troubles, degenerative arthritis, sciatica and constipation. Immune system, reproductive organs and prostate gland |

issues.

**Emotional imbalance:** Being fearful, insecure, needy, nervous and negative. Being stubborn, arrogant, greedy, materialistic, self-centred, angry and violent.

**Unblocking activities:** Walking, martial arts, yoga and other physical activities.

**Cleansing stones:** Ruby, coral, rose quartz, red jasper, garnet, hematite, unakite, bloodstone, tiger's eye and fire agate.

## 2nd Chakra – The Sacral Chakra

| | |
|---|---|
| **Name:** | Sacral Chakra |
| **Sanskrit name:** | Svadhishthana |
| **Sanskrit translation:** | One's own seat or abode |
| **Association:** | Sexuality, creativity and emotions |
| **Meaning:** | I feel |
| **Colour vibration:** | Orange |
| **Element:** | Water |
| **Planet/Star:** | Moon |
| **Gemstone:** | Pearl |
| **Bija mantra:** | VAM |
| **Bija mantra sound:** | V-U-U-U-M-M |
| **Developmental stage:** | From 8 to 14 years old |
| **Location:** | The sacrum. The lower abdomen, around 2 inches below the belly button/ umbilicus at the pelvic plexus. |
| **Cornerstone for self:** | Fluidity, pleasure, healthy sexuality and feeling. |
| **Endocrine glands:** | Reproductive glands (testes in men; ovaries in women); controls sexual development and secretes sex hormones. Blood circulation. |
| **Physical influences:** | Ovaries or testes, prostate, bowel, spleen, large intestine, small intestines, gall bladder, bladder, hips and lower back. |
| **Signs of balance:** | You live a healthy lifestyle, are self-confident, have good physical energy and are well-grounded. You are able to be creative, focused, passionate, sexual, outgoing and take risks. |
| **Physical imbalance:** | Having reproductive, sexual, urinary and kidney problems. Sciatica, chronic |

|                        | lower-back pain and pelvic disorders. |
|------------------------|---------------------------------------|
| **Emotional imbalance:** | Being possessive, jealous, overly promiscuous, insecure, unemotional, closed-off or overly emotional. |
| **Unblocking activities:** | Dancing, belly dancing, stretching, yoga, gardening, moving your hips. Listening to classical music. |
| **Cleansing stones:** | Orange quartz, tiger's eye, coral, orange calcite and jasper. |

## 3rd Chakra – The Solar Plexus Chakra

| | |
|---|---|
| **Name:** | Solar Plexus Chakra |
| **Sanskrit name:** | Manipura |
| **Sanskrit translation:** | Resplendent gem |
| **Association:** | Energy, inner power and will |
| **Meaning:** | I do |
| **Colour vibration:** | Yellow |
| **Element:** | Fire |
| **Planet/Star:** | Jupiter |
| **Gemstone:** | Yellow sapphire |
| **Bija mantra:** | RAM |
| **Bija mantra sound:** | R-U-U-U-M-M |
| **Developmental stage:** | 15 years to 21 years old |
| **Location:** | The solar plexus, between navel and lower ribs, around 3 inches above your belly button. |
| **Cornerstone for self:** | Vitality, spontaneity, willpower, purpose and self-esteem. |
| **Endocrine glands:** | Pancreas; regulates metabolism. |
| **Physical influences:** | Pancreas and digestive system, including the intestines, stomach, gall bladder, liver and middle-upper spine. |
| **Signs of balance:** | You are self-confident, in control, assertive, spontaneous, uninhibited and respectful of others. |
| **Physical imbalance:** | Having problems with your digestion, liver, ulcers or gallstones. Possible issues with anorexia or bulimia, and diabetes or hypoglycaemia. |
| **Emotional imbalance:** | Having a lack of self-esteem, self-confidence, willpower and self-worth. Being fearful, judgemental, controlling, insecure, aggressive and restless. |

**Unblocking activities:** Wearing yellow clothes, having yellow flowers around you, taking some time in the sun and releasing past fears, resentment, worries and anxieties.

**Cleansing stones:** Topaz citrine, tiger's eye, amber, topaz and yellow agate.

## 4th Chakra – The Heart Chakra

| | |
|---|---|
| **Name:** | Heart Chakra |
| **Sanskrit name:** | Anahata |
| **Sanskrit translation:** | Unstruck, Unhurt or Unbeaten |
| **Association:** | Love, Relationships and Healing |
| **Meaning:** | I love |
| **Colour vibration:** | Green (pink outer) |
| **Element:** | Air |
| **Planet/Star:** | Uranus |
| **Gemstone:** | Hessonite |
| **Bija mantra:** | YAM |
| **Bija mantra sound:** | Y-U-U-U-M-M |
| **Developmental stage:** | 22 years to 28 years old |
| **Location:** | In the middle of the sternum, near the heart, in the centre of the chest. |
| **Cornerstone for self:** | Balance, compassion, empathy, self-acceptance, good relationships. |
| **Endocrine glands:** | Thymus gland; regulates the immune system. |
| **Physical influences:** | Heart, lungs, shoulders, arms, ribs, breast, diaphragm, thymus gland, thoracic spine, immune system and circulatory system. |
| **Signs of balance:** | You are compassionate, nurturing, loving, emotionally balanced, friendly, generous and trusting. |
| **Physical imbalance:** | Having problems with heart, lung or blood (AIDS/HIV) diseases, including asthma and bronchial pneumonia. Problems with upper back, ribs, breast, shoulder, arm, wrist and finger pain and high blood pressure. |
| **Emotional imbalance:** | Being jealous, bitter, angry, self-critical, |

|  |  |
|---|---|
|  | resentful, judgemental, possessive, emotionally withheld, cold and distant. Fearful of being alone or rejected. |
| **Unblocking activities:** | Burn Anahata incense and essential oils. Repeat positive affirmations about love. Give and show yourself self-love. Write a journal to express your emotions and feelings. Draw, paint, listen to music or meditate. |
| **Cleansing stones:** | Rose quartz, pink kunzite, emerald, pink tourmaline, jade and malachite. |

## 5th Chakra – The Throat Chakra

| | |
|---|---|
| **Name:** | Throat Chakra |
| **Sanskrit name:** | Vishuddha |
| **Sanskrit translation:** | Pure or purification |
| **Association:** | Communication and truth |
| **Meaning:** | I speak |
| **Colour vibration:** | Blue/sky blue |
| **Element:** | Ether |
| **Planet/Star:** | Mercury |
| **Gemstone:** | Emerald |
| **Bija mantra:** | HAM |
| **Bija mantra sound:** | H-U-U-U-M-M |
| **Developmental stage:** | 29 years to 35 years old |
| **Location:** | The throat – centre, below or around the Adam's apple. |
| **Cornerstone for self:** | Clear communication, creativity and resonance. |
| **Endocrine glands:** | Thyroid gland; regulates body temperature and metabolism. |
| **Physical influences:** | Thyroid and parathyroid glands, throat, vocal cords, mouth, teeth, gums, tongue, oesophagus, tonsils, respiratory system and cervical spine. |
| **Signs of balance:** | You are expressive, honest, truthful, contented, a strong communicator, a good listener, artistic and creative. |
| **Physical imbalance:** | Having problems with the thyroid, sore throats, laryngitis, throat cancer, ear infections, facial issues (chin, lips, tongue, tonsils), mouth and gum ulcers. |
| **Emotional imbalance:** | Being fearful of judgement, ridicule or embarrassment. Unable to express |

yourself in written or spoken word, or unable to speak your truth. Having difficulty communicating, listening to others and lacking in willpower.

**Unblocking activities:** Taking time to meditate or do yoga. Write in a journal or write a poem or song. Singing out loud. Sitting under blue light or lasers. Speaking your truth, especially your hidden truth.

**Cleansing stones:** Blue quartz, blue lace agate, blue topaz and blue lapis.

## 6th Chakra – The Third Eye Chakra

| | |
|---|---|
| **Name:** | Third Eye Chakra |
| **Sanskrit name:** | Ajna |
| **Sanskrit translation:** | Perceive |
| **Association:** | Intuition, vision and imagination |
| **Meaning:** | I see |
| **Colour vibration:** | Indigo |
| **Element:** | All |
| **Planet/Star:** | Venus |
| **Gemstone:** | Diamond |
| **Bija mantra:** | OM or AUM |
| **Bija mantra sound:** | A-U-U-U-M-M |
| **Developmental stage:** | 36 years to 42 years old |
| **Location:** | The centre of the forehead, above the bridge of the nose, behind the middle of your eyebrows. |
| **Cornerstone for self:** | Psychic perception, accurate interpretation, imagination and seeing with clarity. |
| **Endocrine glands:** | Pituitary gland; produces hormones and governs the function of the previous five glands. The pineal gland is also known to be linked with the third eye chakra as well as to the crown chakra. |
| **Physical influences:** | Pituitary and pineal glands, autonomic nervous system, brain, eyes, ears, nose, forehead, face and bones of the skull. |
| **Signs of balance:** | You are focused, determined, charismatic, intuitive, a truth seeker, a puzzle solver, non-materialistic, perceptive and spend most of your time in a state of calm. |

**Physical imbalance:** Having problems with the eyes (blindness), nose (sinus conditions), ears (deafness), brain haemorrhages, brain tumours, seizures, strokes, headaches and learning disabilities.

**Emotional imbalance:** Being indecisive, moody, arrogant, a daydreamer, forgetful, reclusive, difficulty concentrating, having nightmares and hallucinations.

**Unblocking activities:** Using healing crystals separately or together with meditation, reiki, yoga, taking time alone and writing a journal using intuitive thoughts and feelings.

**Cleansing stones:** Sapphire, amethyst, lapis lazuli, fluorite amethyst, charoite and sodalite.

## 7th Chakra – The Crown Chakra

| | |
|---|---|
| **Name:** | Crown Chakra |
| **Sanskrit name:** | Sahasrara |
| **Sanskrit translation:** | Thousand Petals |
| **Association:** | Consciousness and Wisdom |
| **Meaning:** | I understand or I know |
| **Colour vibration:** | Violet |
| **Element:** | All |
| **Planet/Star:** | Neptune |
| **Gemstone:** | Cat's eye |
| **Bija mantra:** | OM or AUM |
| **Bija mantra sound:** | A-U-U-U-M-M (in silence) |
| **Developmental stage:** | 43 to 49 years old |
| **Location:** | The top of the head in the centre, the crown of the head. |
| **Cornerstone for self:** | Wisdom, knowledge, consciousness and spiritual connection. |
| **Endocrine glands:** | Pineal gland; regulates biological cycles, including sleep and wake patterns. |
| **Physical influences:** | Central nervous system, spinal cord, cerebral cortex, brainstem, skull, skeletal system, muscle system and skin. |
| **Signs of balance:** | You are happy within yourself, at peace with yourself, trust in yourself, live in the present moment, aware of greater consciousness and have a magnetic personality. |
| **Physical imbalance:** | Having problems with bone diseases (bone cancer), brain and spinal cord diseases (multiple sclerosis), sensitivity to sound and light, and genetic disorders. |

**Emotional imbalance:** Being depressed, frustrated, indecisive, constant lack of energy, confused, stubborn, lacking focus or direction, sexually confused and overly analytical.

**Unblocking activities:** Taking time to clear and quieten the mind is key, with no phones, electronics, or any possible distractions. Meditation, yoga, reiki, deep breathing, time alone in silence, breathing techniques and silent walks through nature. Connection to everything around you.

**Cleansing stones:** Clear quartz, azeztulite, tanzanite, diamond, amethyst and white jade.

# The 8th And 9th Chakras

Now that we have understood more about the 7 chakras and the connection to our physical bodies, we can now expand our knowledge of chakras to the two most connected chakras outside of our bodies. These chakras are the 8th Chakra (Soul Star Chakra or Soul Chakra) and the 9th Chakra (Stellar Gateway or Gateway Chakra).

These two additional chakras are often discussed using variations of the 9, 12, 13, 16 and 22 chakras systems. They represent energy states that exist outside of our bodies, which is why they sit outside of the 7 chakra system.

Chakras eight and nine are gateways or portals for spiritual purposes and are linked to multidimensional planes. The function of the 8th and 9th chakras is to assist us to be in-tune with multidimensional reality. This includes finding a greater connection to self, receiving energetic healing from the universe, connection to spirit guides, your angels (including your guardian angel) and your spiritual family.

The 8th chakra is often referred to as the energy centre of spiritual compassion, spiritual selflessness and divine love. It is used for connection with our spirit guide and to receive shamanic energetic healing. The 9th chakra extends our connection to allow us to communicate with a variety of spiritual beings including angels, guides and ascended masters.

A number of spiritualists, chakra and meditation specialists and authors on the metaphysical have written that when we die the 8th chakra expands and envelops the 7 chakras of the physical body in a vessel of light, which remains as one until it is time to occupy another body, or vessel.

## 8th Chakra – The Soul Star Chakra

| | |
|---|---|
| **Name:** | Soul Star Chakra |
| **Sanskrit name:** | Vyapini |
| **Sanskrit translation:** | All-pervading or All-encompassing |
| **Association:** | Soul's purpose |
| **Colour vibration:** | Lite ultraviolet (rose) or white/silver light |
| **Element:** | All – The Soul |
| **Planet/Star:** | Saturn |
| **Gemstone:** | Blue sapphire |
| **Location:** | 1-3 inches above your head, outside of the physical body, around an inch above the crown chakra. |
| **Signs of balance:** | You are in control, focused, at peace, completely contented, spiritually aware and connected, at one with the universe and everything in it. |
| **Signs of imbalance:** | Being spaced out, lacking purpose, egotistical, materialistic, lacking energy and lacking direction. No get up and go. |
| **Unblocking activities:** | Meditation, yoga, reiki, deep breathing, time alone in silence, breathing techniques and silent walks through nature. Connection to everything around you. |
| **Cleansing stones:** | Blue kyanite, selenite, Lemurian seed crystal and danburite. |

## 9th Chakra – The Stellar Gateway Chakra

| | |
|---|---|
| **Name:** | Stellar Gateway Chakra |
| **Sanskrit name:** | Vyomanga |
| **Sanskrit translation:** | Universal or Cosmic |
| **Association:** | Devine connection or gateway |
| **Colour vibration:** | Gold |
| **Element:** | All – Spirit – Devine/G-d |
| **Planet/Star:** | Mars |
| **Gemstone:** | Red coral |
| **Location:** | It sits above the physical body and the crown chakra, above the Soul Star chakra, around 6-12 inches above the head. |
| **Signs of balance:** | You are fully at peace with yourself and the world. You have the ability to experience moments of enlightenment. You are living in heaven on earth in your own Lemuria and understand that life is limitless. |
| **Signs of imbalance:** | Being depressed, stubborn in your beliefs, inconsiderate to other opinions, going against yourself, difficulty concentrating and headaches. |
| **Unblocking activities:** | Meditation, yoga, reiki, deep breathing, time alone in silence, breathing techniques and silent walks through nature. |
| **Cleansing stones:** | Azeztulite, moldavite, selenite and stellar beam calcite. |

# Sara Leslie

## International Spiritual Clairvoyant, Medium And Healer

This chapter has been edited with the assistance of Sara Leslie, international spiritual clairvoyant, medium and healer.

Sara Leslie is an internationally recognised professional medium and healer, who specialises in workshops, readings and personalised courses.

If you feel connected by the workings of the metaphysical, including chakras and the spiritual world, contact Sara for a detailed personalised reading.

Use this reference when making contact:
**THE HOLISTIC GUIDE**

Email: saraspirit@hotmail.co.uk

# Numbers Make The World Go Round

*Without mathematics, there's nothing you can do. Everything around you is mathematics. Everything around you is numbers.*
Shakuntala Devi

# Numerology, Your Life Path And The Core Numbers

## What Is Numerology?

Numerology is based on the principle that everything in the universe is connected and that everything is in sync with everything else. Numerology is an ancient metaphysical science that reveals the blueprint of every person's life and abilities.

Numerology takes on two specific roles. First, it is the study of numbers and is seen as a universal language of numbers. Second, using only your full birth name and date of birth, Numerology can be used by anyone to understand more about their own personality, talents, abilities and life events.

Numerology dates back thousands of years to the ancient civilisations of Greece, Egypt, Atlantis, India and Babylon. The Chaldean system of numerology was created in ancient Babylon by the Chaldeans, and is said to be the oldest of all numerology systems created.

It is widely regarded among modern numerologists that the Greek philosopher Pythagoras, born in c.569 BCE, was the father of modern numerology, more than 2,500 years ago. Pythagoras was also considered to be a mathematical genius and the creator of the Pythagorean Theorem. Pythagoras always believed that numbers were far more than just numbers, he believed that each number had an energy, a personality and an identity.

Western Pythagorean numerology is considered to be the most used and accurate system globally today; however, there are still a number of different numerology systems currently being used, including the Chaldeans, Chinese, Kabbalistic and Tamil systems.

## The Basics Of Numerology

Pythagorean Numerology works on the basis that the universe is a system and when individually broken down we are always left with the most basic of elements, which are numbers. This is particularly evident when you take into account the Fibonacci number sequence (1, 1, 2, 3, 5, 8, 13, 21, 34, 55…) and the golden ratio (1.618), which is seen throughout life in the geometry of the human face, the ear (and cochlea), the hand/arm, the body and even DNA. The Fibonacci sequence is also found in trees, plants, flowers and fruits – the spirals in sunflowers and pine cones, the petals on flowers, the lines in the bark of a tree etc.

The Fibonacci sequence is named after Leonardo Pisano (Leonardo of Pisa); he was later dubbed Fibonacci (derived from filius Bonacci – son of Bonacci). Fibonacci was born in Pisa c.1170 and was the first mathematician to introduce Europe to the Hindu-Arabic numerological system with the publication of his *Book of Calculation*, the *Liber Abaci* in 1202.

Pythagoras believed that everything in the universe is mathematically precise, and that each number (letter and symbol) has its own unique vibration and meaning. Numerology shows us that viewing numbers three-dimensionally enables us to see the lessons, guidance and opportunities for personal development within each experience. The way in which the numbers of our date of birth and full birth name (once converted numerologically) are arranged has significant meaning to our lives, personality and desires.

In the Western world today, the Numerologists that are believed to be the authority on the modern methods of numerology include L. Dow Balliett, Matthew Oliver Goodwin, Dr Juno Jordan, David A. Phillips, Hans DeCoz, Michelle Buchanan and Dr Julia Seton.

## Numerology And The Metaphysical

This chapter has been edited with the assistance of Ann Perry, international numerologist. You can find further information on Ann Perry at the end of the chapter.

It has been scientifically proven that everything within our universe has an energy vibration, even down to the smallest of atoms; numbers are exactly the same. Each and every number has its own unique vibration, much like a fingerprint. Numbers are in effect the language of the universe. Humans created the word and the language systems; however, the universe, when broken down into its most simple element, is always left with a number.

If numbers are the language of the universe, it is up to us to become aware and awake enough to take notice and to understand the messages, guidance and communications we are being offered by the universe. This is something we discuss further in the chapter regarding Universal Number messages.

When discussing numerology and its creation, we are always led to the metaphysical world. Numerology is a metaphysical science that dates back thousands of years and is able to reveal the blueprint of every person's life. The reason why numerology is able to do this relates to a deeper understanding of ourselves and our soul's contract, or purpose.

Metaphysically speaking, numerology is based on the fact that every human has a soul within their physical body and will, or has, had many bodies, across many lifetimes. The reason for our soul's incarnation into this life is to learn and evolve through experiences and lessons we encounter within our lives. As we are a collective, the more that we are able to learn individually, the more we are all able to understand as a collective.

Numerology is also based on the understanding that before we incarnate, we sign our soul's contract, choose the vibration of our birth name and choose when we enter the earth plane (each number and letter will carry their own energy and vibration). Before we enter the earth plane, we sign a contract which outlines the lessons and experiences we will have to learn, master and experience throughout this lifetime, this is called our soul's contract. Therefore, by using our date of birth and the given name on our birth certificates, we can ascertain our numerological core numbers, which will give us a greater understanding of ourselves and what lies ahead of us in our lives, including our health, money, career and successes.

Prior to your birth, you would have given a lot of consideration to the vibration of your birth name. You chose the specific vibration of a number because you wanted this number to support your journey within your chosen life path number. Your life path is the lesson you have chosen to learn, while the expression number identifies the talents you have brought with you to support your lesson. Therefore, prior to your birth, you would have sent a telepathic message to whomever would name you in this lifetime. You would have said: 'I do not care what name you call me. Call me whatever you like. However! Make sure my name vibrates at the specific vibration of my chosen number, because that is what I have chosen to support me on this journey.' The person will pick up on this vibe and name the child accordingly.

Within numerology, the guidance and life blueprint given describes your life's energy pattern, similar to that of a weather pattern. As with a weather report, it only gives guidance to the weather patterns without facts. With the weather, it could, might, should be rainy, sunny, windy etc. The same applies with a numerology blueprint, it gives you the energies around you at a given time, and your personality influences. It does not provide the specifics of everyday life as each number holds both positive and negative energies that must be harnessed for its full utilisation.

This is why it is possible that a person may not connect or resonate with their numerology blueprint, especially when looking forward in time. When looking into the past, it is possible that numerology can validate your past experiences, as well as giving comfort and understanding to the lessons within those experiences.

Numerology and numbers are very clear, very practical and very precise. Numbers only work in facts, and numerology is there to decipher the energies and vibrations within our soul's code (our date of birth and given name on our birth certificates) and within the letters, symbols and numbers in our world.

## The Chakra-Numerology Connection

As we have already discussed in this chapter, everything in life is connected in some way, chakras and numerology are no different with some very visible and obvious overlaps. When looking into the translation or meaning of the numbers 1 to 9, take a closer look at the colour reference between the chakra's colour vibration and the vibration of the number colour, they are always the same. Additionally, chakras and numbers are also linked by having the same gemstone and planet association.

Every number within numerology relates to both positive and negative characteristics. These can be associated with personality, guidance or warnings. By using our knowledge of chakras from this book, we are able to balance ourselves, unblock our chakras and bring forward the positive energies that are associated with these numbers.

When we are able to freely open ourselves up and unblock our chakras, we become far more balanced, considered and at peace with ourselves and the universe. This in turn allows us to expand and emphasise the positive energies of the numbers that are connected within our own numerology chart.

There are nine numbers and nine major chakras, with each one having a cause and effect on the other, with the understanding from the previous chapter that chakras are the energy transducers for subtle energy, and that numbers in our numerology chart have their own unique energy. It is therefore possible, if not likely, that chakras are not only energy transducers for subtle energy, they are also the energy transducers for the energy of numbers in the universe and our numerology chart, which are also likely to be subtle energies.

## How Can Numerology Improve Your Life?

Numerology is a wonderful self-help tool that has many benefits when used throughout your life, not to mention the most obvious, having your life map available to you for guidance and understanding. This is a true gift of insight.

For many people, numerology has the ability to give life meaning, an understanding that there are no random events and that everything happens for a reason. Everything in your life happens for you and for your soul's benefit to achieve its predestined life purpose. Here are some other ways that numerology can improve your life:

- Numerology can show you your life map or blueprint
- Numerology can assist you in understanding yourself with greater understanding and deeper meaning
- Numerology can give you clarity on your predestined life path
- Numerology can give you an understanding of how others see you
- Numerology can help you uncover your full potential in your life
- Numerology can uncover the true and authentic you
- Numerology can give you an understanding of your own talents and abilities
- Numerology can give you the ability to fully understand the events that have taken place in your life
- Numerology can help you plan for a major life event
- Numerology can prepare you for what may lie ahead in your future
- Numerology can give you the confidence you require to know you are on the right path in your life
- Numerology can give you a direction to follow in your life

- Numerology can help validate past situations or events
- Numerology can assist in choosing the 'numerologically right day' for any situation
- Numerology can assist you in choosing the right career path or job move
- Numerology can help in choosing a suitable partner, either business or love partner
- Numerology can help strengthen relationships and assess compatibility
- Numerology can assist you in understanding others and their actions
- Numerology can give you confidence in exploring opportunities that arise
- Numerology can help with choosing a baby name, a company name or the address of your home
- Numerology can give you the ability to fully understand yourself
- Numerology can assist you in understanding and deciphering the meaning of recurring numbers (for more information go to page 227 for The Universal Number Messages)

# The Numerology Core Numbers

For the purposes of this book, and an introduction into numerology, we are focusing on the five core numerology numbers that assist in the make-up of your talents, personality and life blueprint. As a rule of thumb, anything that comes from the date of birth is typically a lesson, and anything that comes from the birth name reveals talents, gifts and passions.

## *Life Path Number*

Within the five core numbers in numerology, the Life Path Number, also referred to as the Birth Force or Lesson Number, is the most important and valuable number. The Life Path Number provides important and detailed information about your personality, the life you will live, experiences you will encounter and lessons you are destined to learn.

## *Expression Or Destiny Number*

The Expression Number, or Destiny Number, is one of the most important core numbers in numerology; it is in fact the second most important number behind the Life Path. The Expression Number reveals your character, personality, abilities and talents. This number guides you to what you are destined to do in this lifetime and who you will become.

## *Heart's Desire Or Soul's Urge Number*

The Heart's Desire Number, or Soul's Urge Number, is the third most significant number in the numerology chart and reveals the inner you, the real you, the you very few people will ever see. It reveals all of your hopes, dreams, wishes, passions and desires.

The Heart's Desire Number also tells of your soul's talents, whether these are active, dormant or progressed in this life.

## Personality Number

The Personality Number, or Outer You Number, is said to be the least significant of the core numbers. The Personality Number reveals the 'outer you', the you that is projected onto the world and discloses how other people perceive you. This is your outer shell that the world sees and not how you think, feel or see yourself.

## Birth Day Number

The Birth Day Number is aligned with the Life Path Number and can be referred to as a 'sub-lesson' to the main lessons of the Life Path Number. The Birth Day Number highlights those special talents within your capabilities that will help and progress you through life's journey.

## The Other Numerology Numbers

While I have focused on the five core numerology numbers, there are many other numerology numbers that can offer additional insight into your character, motivation, talents and purpose. These include:

- Achievement Number
- Ancestral Traits Number
- Balance Number
- Hidden Passion Number
- Inner Talents Number
- Karmic Debt Number
- Life Lessons Number

- Personal Day Number
- Personal Month Number
- Personal Year Number

# The Methods Of Numerology

Within numerology there are differing methods of calculating the numbers. It is the belief of many numerologists, myself and Ann Perry included, that there is only one way that ensures you are receiving all the relevant information available from your numbers, including the sub-lessons.

There are two main methods of calculating numerology numbers, the Straight-Across, or Straight-Line, Method; and the method outlined in the chapters below, let's call this the Complete Method.

I have adopted this method for a number of reasons. When we add up all the numbers in a date of birth using the straight-line method, it does not allow the birth 'day' number to stand out as its own core number. This number has significant value to interpreting someone's birth code. However, the more important reason for using the Complete Method is that when you add the numbers straight across you will often bring up incorrect sub-lessons relating to the life path number.

### *Straight-Across Method Example – Life Path Number*

- Using your full date of birth (DD/MM/YYYY)
- Add up all the numbers of your date of birth (DD/MM/YYYY)
- Adding each day, month and year number together
- Keep adding until you get an 11, 22, 33, 44...or a single digit. Numbers 11, 22, 33, 44...are NOT to be reduced to a single number as these are Master Numbers
- Then add all the numbers for each together until you get an 11, 22, 33, 44...or a single digit

## Straight-Across Method Example Continued

For example, if your date of birth was 25 March 1959, 25/03/1959, the following would be true using the straight-line method:
Added straight across it would look like this:

**Total** – 2 + 5 + 0 + 3 + 1 + 9 + 5 + 9 = **34**

**Example Life Path Number** – 3 + 4 = 7

This would mean that this person's Life Path Number is a 7 (34/7) and their sub-lessons would be a 3 (learning how to express themselves creatively) and the 4 (learning about planning, process and discipline) so they can be the best 7 they can be.

## Complete Method Example – Life Path Number

Using the Complete Method, as detailed below, will bring through clear and accurate sub-lessons.

- Using your full date of birth (DD/MM/YYYY)
- Add up all the numbers of your date of birth (DD/MM/YYYY)
- Adding each day, month and year number individually
- Keep adding until you get an 11, 22, 33, 44…or a single digit. Numbers 11, 22, 33, 44…are NOT to be reduced to a single number as these are Master Numbers
- Then add all the numbers for each together until you get an 11, 22, 33, 44…or a single digit

## Complete Method Example Continued

For example, if your date of birth was 25 March 1959, 25/03/1959, the following would be true using the complete method:

The day, 25, is reduced to:

2 + 5 = **7**

The month, 03, is reduced to:

0 + 3 = **3**

The year, 1959, is reduced to:

1 + 9 + 5 + 9 = **24**

(24) 2 + 4 = **6**

**Total** – 3 + 7 + 6 = **16**

**Example Life Path Number** – 1 + 6 = 7

Now we see entirely different sub-lessons associated with the life path number of 7 (16/7). We see a 1 (learning how to be an independent, creative leader) and the 6 (learning lessons related to responsibility and perfectionism) to be the best 7 they can be.

## Our Method Conclusion

Ann and I both believe that when we simply reduce the numbers using the straight-across method, it can be less beneficial than it is possible for it to be and therefore we can receive either incomplete or incorrect information. That being said, the only way to know which sub-lessons relate to you is to do the calculations both ways. When you have both sets of calculations, you can assess which one 'feels' and resonates more in alignment with you and your life journey.

There is no way to prove which system is correct; however,

utilising Ann's years of experience examining people's charts (while discussing the results with them), and my own knowledge, has led me to believe that the date of birth must be broken down independently if you wish to have a more accurate understanding of the sub-lessons.

# How To Calculate Your Core Numerology Numbers

At this stage of the book, this is your opportunity to pause for a moment and work through your own core numerology numbers. When you have calculated your own numbers, you can then use them to relate the information in this chapter to you, your personality and your life path.

### Your Life Path Number

The Life Path number is the LESSON number and representative of your journey through this lifetime. This is where you will find all of the lessons you agreed to learn prior to your incarnation. It highlights specific elements of our personality, talents, potential and reveals our greater purpose.

The Life Path Number is derived from your date of birth, by adding all of the numerical values in your full date of birth.

### *How To Calculate Your Life Path Number*

- Using your full date of birth (DD/MM/YYYY)
- Add up all the numbers of your date of birth (DD/MM/YYYY)
- Adding each day, month and year number individually
- Keep adding until you get an 11, 22, 33, 44...or a single digit. Numbers 11, 22, 33, 44...are NOT to be reduced to a single number as these are Master Numbers
- Then add all the numbers for each together until you get an 11, 22, 33, 44...or a single digit

## *Life Path Number Example*

Basketball legend Michael Jordan, born Michael Jeffrey Jordan, has his birthday on 17 February 1963, 17/02/1963; therefore the following is true for his Life Path Number:

The day, 17, is reduced to:
1 + 7 = **8**

The month, 02, is reduced to:
0 + 2 = **2**

The year, 1963, is reduced to:
1 + 9 + 6 + 3 = **19**
(19) 1 + 9 = **10**
(10) 1 + 0 = **1**

**Total** – 8 + 2 + 1 = **11 (2)**

Michael Jordan's Life Path Number is 11; this is also connected to the number 2.

## *Calculate Your Life Path Number*

Use the space below to work out your Life Path Number.

Your Day of birth:

Your Month of birth:

Your Year of birth:

Your Life Path Number:

# Your Expression Number

The Expression or Destiny Number illuminates the gifts, talents and abilities you chose to support you on your life's journey. These can assist in understanding certain situations or help in making wiser and more astute decisions. The Expression Number comes from the name you were given at birth, by adding the numerical values of all the letters in your given name.

## *How To Calculate Your Expression Number*

Use the Pythagorean numerology chart below, which is there to give a numerical value to each letter of the alphabet:

| | | | | |
|---|---|---|---|---|
| **1** | = | A | J | S |
| **2** | = | B | K | T |
| **3** | = | C | L | U |
| **4** | = | D | M | V |
| **5** | = | E | N | W |
| **6** | = | F | O | X |
| **7** | = | G | P | Y |
| **8** | = | H | Q | Z |
| **9** | = | I | R | |

- Using your full birth name (first, middle, last)
- Transfer the letters in your name into numbers using the Pythagorean chart above
- Adding the first, middle and surnames up individually
- Keep adding until you get an 11, 22, 33, 44…or a single digit. Numbers 11, 22, 33, 44…are NOT to be reduced to a single number as these are Master Numbers
- Then add all the numbers for each together until you get an 11, 22, 33, 44…or a single digit

## *Expression Number Example*

The 42nd President of the United States of America was Bill Clinton. His full birth name is William Jefferson Blythe, therefore the following is true for his Expression Number:

W + I + L + L + I + A + M
5 + 9 + 3 + 3 + 9 + 1 + 4 = **34**
(34) 3 + 4 = **7**

J + E + F + F + E + R + S + O + N
1 + 5 + 6 + 6 + 5 + 9 + 1 + 6 + 5 = **44**

B + L + Y + T + H + E
2 + 3 + 7 + 2 + 8 + 5 = **27**
(27) 2 + 7 = **9**

**Total** – 7 + 44 + 9 = **60**
(60) 6 + 0 = **6**

Bill Clinton's Expression Number is 6.

*Calculate Your Expression Number*

Your First Name:

Your Middle Name:

Your Last Name:

Your Expression Number:

# Your Heart's Desire Number

The Heart's Desire or Soul's Urge Number is a reflection of your inner true self and what it is that you truly want and are passionate about: your heart's desire. Being in touch and at one with our authentic self is the best way to fulfil our heart's desire, and to succeed in being the best version of ourselves.

The Heart's Desire Number comes from the name you were given at birth, by adding the numerical values of the VOWELS in your given name.

## *How To Calculate Your Heart's Desire Number*

- Using your full birth name (first, middle, last), use only the VOWELS in each name
- Remember that Y or W are not used as vowels, only A, E, I, O and U (other methods can include these)
- Transfer the letters in your name into numbers using the Pythagorean chart above
- Adding the VOWELS in your first, middle and surnames up individually
- Keep adding until you get an 11, 22, 33, 44…or a single digit. Numbers 11, 22, 33, 44…are NOT to be reduced to a single number as these are Master Numbers
- Then add all the numbers for each together until you get an 11, 22, 33, 44…or a single digit

## *Heart's Desire Number Example*

Known by most as the King of Pop, Michael Jackson was born Michael Joseph Jackson, therefore the following is true for his Heart's Desire Number:

M + **I** + C + H + **A** + **E** + L
0 + 9 + 0 + 0 + 1 + 5 = **15**
(15) 1 + 5 = **6**

J + **O** + S + **E** + P + H
0 + 6 + 0 + 5 + 0 + 0 = **11**

J + **A** + C + K + S + **O** + N
0 + 1 + 0 + 0 + 0 + 6 = **7**

**Total** – 6 + 11 + 7 = **24**
(24) 2 + 4 = **6**

Michael Jackson's Heart's Desire Number is 6.

## *Calculate Your Heart's Desire Number*

Your First Name:

Your Middle Name:

Your Last Name:

Your Heart's Desire Number:

# Your Personality Number

The Personality Number is there to give greater clarity and understanding to your own personality. It can also reveal greater insights into your own patterns of behaviour in circumstances or situations.

The Personality Number comes from the name you were given at birth by adding the numerical values of the CONSONANTS in your given name.

## *How To Calculate Your Personality Number*

- Using your full birth name (first, middle, last), use only the CONSONANTS in each name
- Transfer the letters in your name into numbers using the Pythagorean chart above
- Adding the CONSONANTS in your first, middle and surnames up individually
- Keep adding until you get an 11, 22, 33, 44…or a single digit. Numbers 11, 22, 33, 44…are NOT to be reduced to a single number as these are Master Numbers
- Then add all the numbers for each together until you get an 11, 22, 33, 44…or a single digit

## *Personality Number Example*

Former president of South Africa, Nelson Mandela; his full birth name is Nelson Rolihlahla Mandela, therefore the following is true for his Personality Number:

**N + E + L + S + O + N**
5 + 0 + 3 + 1 + 0 + 5 = **14**
(14) 1 + 4 = **5**

**R + O + L + I + H + L + A + H + L + A**
9 + 0 + 3 + 0 + 8 + 3 + 0 + 8 + 3 + 0 = **34**
(34) 3 + 4 = **7**

**M + A + N + D + E + L + A**
4 + 0 + 5 + 4 + 0 + 3 + 0 = **16**
(16) 1 + 6 = **7**

**Total** – 5 + 7 + 7 = **19**
(19) 1 + 9 = **10**
(10) 1 + 0 = **1**

Nelson Mandela's Personality Number is 1.

## *Calculate Your Personality Number*

Your First Name:

Your Middle Name:

Your Last Name:

Your Personality Number:

# Your Birth Day Number

The Birth Day Number can reveal any specific talents or abilities you possess. As one of the five core numbers in numerology, the Birth Day Number also gives an insight into who you are and your ability to influence life situations.

The Birth Day Number is derived from your date of birth, by adding the numerical values in your day of birth.

## *How To Calculate Your Birth Day Number*

- Using the day ONLY of birth (DD)
- Add up the numbers of your day of birth (DD)
- Keep adding until you get an 11, 22, 33, 44...or a single digit. Numbers 11, 22, 33, 44...are NOT to be reduced to a single number as these are Master Numbers
- Then add all the numbers for each together until you get an 11, 22, 33, 44...or a single digit

## *Birth Day Number Example*

World renowned physicist Albert Einstein's birthday was 14 March 1879, 14/03/1879, therefore the following is true for his Birth Day Number:

The day, 14, is reduced to:
1 + 4 = **5**

Albert Einstein's Birth Day Number is 5.

## *Calculate Your Birth Day Number*

Your Day of Birth:

Your Birth Day Number:

## *Your Core Numerology Numbers*

Once you have calculated your core numerology numbers, keep a note of them below. This will assist you in interpreting the numbers in the following chapter. Initially, it is recommended that you focus on your own core numerology numbers before turning your attention to family and friends.

Life Path Number:

Expression Number:

Heart's Desire Number:

Personality Number:

Birth Day Number:

# What Do The Numbers Mean?

## Understanding The Numerology Meanings

As we have already touched on, each and every number has its own energy vibration and connectivity. In this chapter we are focusing on the meanings, traits and personalities behind each of the numbers, one to nine.

As we understand what numbers we are connected with ourselves, we can use these sections as guidance for our life, career, relationships etc., as well as giving us an understanding of our personality, goals, dreams and aspirations.

According to author and researcher Brian Baulsom, who has over 40 years of practical astrology and tarot experience, odd numbers are masculine and even numbers are feminine. This is not the gender specific version of masculine and feminine, these are the specific personality traits of the energy within the numbers and therefore around and within us all.

**Masculine** – active, creative, forward/aggressive and cold
**Feminine** – passive, receptive, yielding and warm

## Keywords Connected To The Numbers

| | | |
|---|---|---|
| **Number 1** | – | Leader |
| **Number 2** | – | Peacekeeper |
| **Number 3** | – | Communicator |
| **Number 4** | – | Planner |
| **Number 5** | – | Freedom seeker |
| **Number 6** | – | Nurturer |
| **Number 7** | – | Analyst |
| **Number 8** | – | Business leader |
| **Number 9** | – | Humanitarian |

# What Does It All Mean?

**Planet/Star:** the planet/star the number is associated with.

**Element:** the earthly element the number is associated with.

**Colour vibration:** the colour of the vibration from the number's energy or the energy radiating from the number.

**Gemstone:** the gemstone the number is associated with.

**Top strengths:** the personality strengths the number is associated with in your numerology chart.

**Top challenges:** the personality challenges the number is associated with in your numerology chart.

**Be wary:** be wary of these personality traits if you have this number in your numerology chart.

**Guidance:** guidance for those with this number in their numerology chart.

**Career:** career guidance for those with this number in their numerology chart.

# Number 1

## The Leader – The Independent Person

Number 1 on an individual basis is often saved for those with a pioneering spirit and leadership capabilities. The 1 is here to learn how to be independent rather than being dependent.

| | |
|---|---|
| **Planet/Star:** | Sun |
| **Element:** | Fire |
| **Colour vibration:** | Red |
| **Gemstone:** | Ruby |

| | |
|---|---|
| **Top Strengths:** | Pioneering |
| | Courageous |
| | Innovative |
| | Self-motivated |
| | Determined |

| | |
|---|---|
| **Top Challenges:** | Impatient |
| | Intolerant |
| | Controlling |
| | Competitive |
| | Aggressive |

**Be Wary** – you be can be boastful, demanding, impatient, stubborn, critical, self-centred, single-minded and lonely.

**Guidance** – do not forget those around you; you need them for support, even if you do not think so.

**Career** – a truthful and honest leader, entrepreneur, visionary or storyteller.

**Masculine** – active, creative, forward/aggressive and cold.

## *Life Path – Number 1*

As a Life Path Number 1, you will have many of the following lessons to learn and work through in your lifetime.

### *The Life Lessons*

- You are to learn to be the decision-maker in most relationships and partnerships
- You are to learn to be a great leader
- You are to learn to be focused on your specific goals
- You are to learn that the sky is the limit
- You are to learn to never give up
- You are to learn to be determined and courageous
- You are to learn to be a pioneer
- You are to learn to take risks
- You are to learn to be an unstoppable force
- You are to learn to have a strong sense of integrity
- You are to learn to be practical
- You are to learn to be creative
- You are to learn to use your natural creativity
- You are to learn to be ambitious in promoting yourself
- You are to learn to be at the forefront
- You are to learn to be action-orientated
- You are to learn to be self-sufficient
- You are to learn to forge your own path
- You are to learn a strong sense of right and wrong
- You are to learn to be unafraid of confrontation
- You are to learn to either work alone or lead a team
- You are to learn not to be selfish and self-centred
- You are to learn not to be a follower
- You are to learn not to be domineering
- You are to learn not to be egotistical
- You are to learn not to waste time

## *Expression – Number 1*

As an Expression Number 1, you chose to bring with you these talents and gifts to support your chosen Life Path Number.

- You are a pioneer
- You are a risk-taker
- You are someone who puts themselves out on a limb
- You are someone who enjoys trying new things
- You are independent
- You are self-sufficient
- You are highly opinionated
- You are extremely capable in your field of choice
- You are a natural leader
- You are someone who takes charge, even in the unknown
- You are result-orientated
- You are highly ambitious
- You are usually one of the trendsetters

## *Heart's Desire – Number 1*

As a Heart's Desire Number 1, you chose to bring with you these talents, gifts and passions to illuminate your life's purpose.

- You have a desire for independence and leadership
- You have a desire to be creative
- You have a desire to be action-orientated
- You have a desire to be confident in your own judgements
- You have a desire to be a strong leader, with followers
- You have a desire to be independent and self-sufficient
- You have a desire to live life to the full and try new things
- You have a desire for great success
- You have a desire to be in complete control of your destiny
- You have a desire to have no issues making bold, daring and controversial decisions, when you are convinced in yourself
- You have a desire to forge your own path based on your beliefs and principles

## *Personality – Number 1*

As a Personality Number 1, you will have many of the following personality traits in your life.

- You are confident
- You are forward thinking
- You are independent
- You are focused
- You are a natural leader
- You are creative
- You are practical
- You are honest
- You are impassioned
- You are action-orientated
- You are not a time waster
- You are loyal
- You are ambitious

## *Birth Day – Number 1*

As a Birth Day Number 1, you will have many of the following traits and focuses in your life.

- You have a desire for individuality
- Your ambitions drive and motivate you
- You have a strong motivation to succeed in life
- You function well independently
- Routine bores and frustrates you
- Leadership is natural to you
- You are comfortable being a pioneer or innovator
- You are a knowledge seeker
- You are loyal and honest
- You are creative
- You are practical
- You prefer not to deal with the frustrations and limitations of having to work with others

# Number 2

## The Peacekeeper – The Co-Operator

Number 2 brings with it diplomacy, intuition and guidance, those who can guide with a soft hand and rule with a strong arm and iron will. The 2 is here to learn how to be a team player rather than a passive observer.

| | |
|---|---|
| **Planet/Star:** | Moon |
| **Element:** | Water |
| **Colour vibration:** | Orange |
| **Gemstone:** | Pearl |
| | |
| **Top Strengths:** | Harmonious |
| | Intuitive |
| | Loving |
| | Supportive |
| | Understanding |
| | |
| **Top Challenges:** | Moody |
| | Hypersensitive |
| | Insecure |
| | Jealous |
| | Indecisive |

**Be Wary** – you can be overly sensitive, can feel unappreciated, can over-cooperate and be subservient.

**Guidance** – you need balance. It is good to help people; however, set healthy boundaries and say 'no' when you need to. Do not forget about you.

**Career** – you are a writer, peacemaker and work well in a team. Look at roles in teaching or as a caregiver.

**Feminine** – passive, receptive, yielding and warm.

## *Life Path – Number 2*

As a Life Path Number 2, you will have many of the following lessons to learn and work through in your lifetime.

## *The Life Lessons*

- You are to learn to be continually balanced and fair
- You are to learn to be gentle and loyal
- You are to learn to be patient
- You are to learn to be kind and loving
- You are to learn to be a great listener
- You are to learn to take the role of leader
- You are to learn to be a guide and teacher to others
- You are to learn to be diplomatic and peace-loving
- You are to learn to avoid confrontation at all costs
- You are to learn to use your natural sensitivity
- You are to learn to interact with others
- You are to learn to be all sides of a situation or discussion
- You are to learn to work behind the scenes
- You are to learn to rarely be in the limelight
- You are to learn to use your well-liked personality
- You are to learn to have a sincere concern for others
- You are to learn to see the best of people
- You are to learn to be honest in thought, word and deed
- You are to learn to please and serve others
- You are to learn to have the ability to say 'No'
- You are to learn to keep your anger in check when crossed
- You are to learn to use your great passion for music
- You are to learn not to be overly demanding
- You are to learn not to blame others for wrongdoings
- You are to learn not to come across as shy
- You are to learn not to be overprotective
- You are to learn not to be indecisive

## *Expression – Number 2*

As an Expression Number 2, you chose to bring with you these talents and gifts to support your chosen Life Path Number.

- You are very expressive and outgoing
- You are relatable to many different people
- You are a strong communicator
- You are a natural charmer
- You are a harmonious and peaceful person
- You are nurturing and empathetic
- You are someone who avoids confrontation
- You are intuitive and can often feel others' feelings
- You are someone who works best as part of a team
- You are naturally patient
- You are supportive
- You are diplomatic
- You are connected with the arts (acting, music, writing)
- You are someone who has natural rhythm and harmony

## *Heart's Desire – Number 2*

As a Heart's Desire Number 2, you chose to bring with you these talents, gifts and passions to illuminate your life's purpose.

- You have a desire to be a peacekeeper
- You have a desire to bridge gaps and resolve disputes
- You have a desire to bring others together in cooperation
- You have a desire to be diplomatic
- You have a desire for peace and harmony
- You have a desire to achieve the perfect balance in life
- You have a desire to seek comfort and desire partnerships
- You have a desire to fall in love rather easily
- You have a desire to shy away from conflict
- You have a desire to appreciate the finer things in life
- You have a desire to want a refined sense of taste
- You have a desire to have a talent and passion for music

## *Personality – Number 2*

As a Personality Number 2, you will have many of the following traits and focuses in your life.

- You are loving
- You are intuitive
- You are charismatic
- You are harmonious
- You are peaceful
- You are diplomatic
- You are trustworthy
- You are open-minded
- You are unpretentious
- You are balanced
- You are artistic
- You are expressive
- You are musical
- You are hypersensitive

## *Birth Day – Number 2*

As a Birth Day Number 2, you will have many of the following traits and focuses in your life.

- You appreciate balance and peace
- You have the ability to be an inspirational team player
- You have a passion for the arts, beauty and nature
- You have a desire for partnerships
- Affection from those close to you is important
- You can be naturally affected by your surroundings
- You have a strong understanding of people
- You are loyal, honest and trustworthy
- You prefer to be surrounded by peace and harmony
- You are highly intuitive of others
- You can be overly sensitive and hurt easily
- You can lack confidence

# Number 3

## The Communicator – The Entertainer

Number 3 is a strong and positive number. Those associated with the number 3 are usually the life of the party and believe that the world is full of wonder and opportunity. The 3 is here to be an upbeat communicator rather than someone who berates themselves and their talents.

| | |
|---|---|
| **Planet/Star:** | Jupiter |
| **Element:** | Fire |
| **Colour vibration:** | Yellow |
| **Gemstone:** | Yellow Sapphire |
| | |
| **Top Strengths:** | Humorous |
| | Imaginative |
| | Creative |
| | Friendly |
| | Charismatic |
| | |
| **Top Challenges:** | Scattered |
| | Critical |
| | Melodramatic |
| | Attention-seeking |
| | Gossipy |

**Be Wary** – you can be self-conscious, hide your emotions and can be withdrawn.

**Guidance** – protect yourself at all times and trust who you are to be at one with yourself. Speak your truth.

**Career** – you are a social person and a team player with a positive attitude. A position in sales, a politician or in mediation.

**Masculine** – active, creative, forward, aggressive and cold.

## *Life Path – Number 3*

As a Life Path Number 3, you will have many of the following lessons to learn and work through in your lifetime.

## *The Life Lessons*

- You are to learn to love communicating with people
- You are to learn to enjoy connecting with people
- You are to learn to be naturally warm and friendly
- You are to learn to love living life
- You are to learn to enjoy every day
- You are to learn to appreciate the beauty of the world
- You are to learn to share your ideas and feelings
- You are to learn to be a breath of fresh air for people
- You are to learn to be young at heart
- You are to learn to be very expressive
- You are to learn to enjoy all of art as an expressive tool
- You are to learn to be charismatic
- You are to learn to be charming
- You are to learn to be a talented entertainer
- You are to learn to be a strong conversationalist
- You are to learn to be an intuitive listener
- You are to learn to be positive by nature
- You are to learn to be a giver rather than a taker
- You are to learn to settle in one place
- You are to learn to take time to mature
- You are to learn not to become moody without reasoning
- You are to learn not to lack self-discipline
- You are to learn not to be distracted easily
- You are to learn not to leave situations/projects unfinished
- You are to learn not to procrastinate
- You are to learn not to be deeply insecure and critical
- You are to learn not to hide your emotions and feelings

## *Expression – Number 3*

As an Expression Number 3, you chose to bring with you these talents and gifts to support your chosen Life Path Number.

- You are naturally theatrical
- You are outgoing and expressive
- You are someone who has a positive personality and outlook
- You are someone with an interest in writing, acting or the arts
- You are a great translator and communicator
- You are someone who is charismatic and charming
- You are able to inspire others with ease
- You are someone with infectious enthusiasm
- You are someone with a great sense of humour
- You are someone with a constant creative streak
- You are quick-witted
- You are materialistic
- You are harsh and blunt

## *Heart's Desire – Number 3*

As a Heart's Desire Number 3, you chose to bring with you these talents, gifts and passions to illuminate your life's purpose.

- You have a desire to be a naturally friendly person
- You have a desire to have creative talents
- You have a desire to be a natural entertainer
- You have a desire to be intuitive
- You have a desire to be mentally and emotionally balanced
- You have a desire to be inspirational
- You have a desire to be a great communicator
- You have a desire to have a talent for natural expression
- You have a desire to inspire people with your personality
- You have a desire to be an outgoing person
- You have a desire to be eloquent
- You have a desire to be playful and joyous
- You have a desire to be able to express your feelings

## *Personality – Number 3*

As a Personality Number 3, you will have many of the following traits and focuses in your life.

- You are charming
- You are positive
- You are extroverted
- You are charismatic
- You are a great communicator
- You are optimistic
- You are magnetically beautiful
- You are someone who loves to love
- You are creative
- You are inspirational
- You are judgemental
- You are very critical
- You are materialistic

## *Birth Day – Number 3*

As a Birth Day Number 3, you will have many of the following traits and focuses in your life.

- You have a need to express yourself
- You can be charming and inspirational
- You enjoy being sociable
- You have a loving nature
- You are quick-witted
- You are eloquent
- You are very creative and imaginative
- You have an enthusiasm for life
- You can lack discipline and focus
- You can be emotionally up and down
- You can be materialistic
- You are likely to be a success within the fields of writing, music, performing or visual arts

# Number 4

## The Planner – The Worker

There is no grey scale related to Number 4, it is either black or white. This number is connected with being blunt, honest and direct. Being organised and following orders is a key personality trait for a number 4.

| | |
|---|---|
| **Planet/Star:** | Uranus |
| **Element:** | Earth |
| **Colour vibration:** | Green |
| **Gemstone:** | Hessonite |
| | |
| **Top Strengths:** | Hard working |
| | Organised |
| | Grounded |
| | Responsible |
| | Focused |
| | |
| **Top Challenges:** | Inflexible |
| | Intolerant |
| | Stubborn |
| | Narrow-minded |
| | Pessimistic |

**Be Wary** – you can be stubborn and too rigid. You need to find balance in your life.

**Guidance** – believe in yourself, follow your intuition and take a leap of faith.

**Career** – you are organised and disciplined. Chief Operating Officer, event planner, military or engineering are good professions for you.

**Feminine** – passive, receptive, yielding and warm.

## *Life Path – Number 4*

As a Life Path Number 4, you will have many of the following lessons to learn and work through in your lifetime.

### *The Life Lessons*

- You are to learn to be hard working
- You are to learn to have a strong work ethic
- You are to learn to be results-driven
- You are to learn to have success in business
- You are to learn to be an excellent manager
- You are to learn to be a traditionalist
- You are to learn to have a strong sense of morality
- You are to learn to be loyal
- You are to learn to be mentally strong
- You are to learn to be direct and honest
- You are to learn to see life in black or white, no grey
- You are to learn to be dedicated to your work
- You are to learn to be very organised
- You are to learn to be dependable and reliable
- You are to learn to be emotionally stable
- You are to learn to be grounded
- You are to learn to be a good provider
- You are to learn to complete tasks for others who struggle
- You are to learn to have a sense of tradition and morality
- You are to learn to have a high level of integrity
- You are to learn to have a balanced and stable environment
- You are to learn to be devoted to family and friends
- You are to learn not to be judgemental
- You are to learn not to be frustrated by limitations
- You are to learn not to lack creatively
- You are to learn not to be intolerant and stubborn
- You are to learn not to be controlling

## *Expression – Number 4*

As an Expression Number 4, you chose to bring with you these talents and gifts to support your chosen Life Path Number.

- You are down-to-earth
- You are practical and structured
- You are seen as a pillar of strength for others
- You are disciplined and dutiful
- You are a dedicated worker
- You are someone with an orderly nature
- You are someone who takes your responsibilities seriously
- You are trustworthy with integrity
- You are loyal and honest
- You are reliable and dependable
- You are stubborn
- You are judgemental
- You are too focused on rules and regulations

## *Heart's Desire – Number 4*

As a Heart's Desire Number 4, you chose to bring with you these talents, gifts and passions to illuminate your life's purpose.

- You have a desire to be loyal and honest
- You have a desire to be driven by results
- You have a desire to be a success in business
- You have a desire to be reliable and dependable
- You have a desire to be an achiever
- You have a desire to be analytical
- You have a desire to be focused on your work
- You have a desire to be logical
- You have a desire to enjoy routine
- You have a desire to be organised
- You have a desire to be ethical
- You have a desire to be flexible and adaptable
- You have a desire to be family focused

## *Personality – Number 4*

As a Personality Number 4, you will have many of the following traits and focuses in your life.

- You are honest
- You are blunt
- You are hard working
- You are loyal
- You are detail-orientated
- You are reliable
- You are dependable
- You are balanced
- You are disciplined
- You are logical
- You are mentally strong
- You are family focused
- You are stubborn

## *Birth Day – Number 4*

As a Birth Day Number 4, you will have many of the following traits and focuses in your life.

- You have a need to plan
- You love to organise
- You are reliable and dependable
- You have a strong focus on your work life
- You like tradition and have traditional values
- You are naturally logical and practical
- You have your feet firmly on the ground
- You take pride in what you have achieved
- You are ethical
- You are mentally strong
- You are conscientious
- You can be rigid in your focus
- You can lack creativity due to narrow-mindedness

# Number 5

## The Adventurer – The Freedom Seeker

Those associated with the number 5 are often described as footloose and fancy-free, or free-spirited. They do not like to be tied down to commitments and are always the first ready for a new adventure. The 5 is here to learn how to use their freedom in constructive ways rather than scattering their energy.

| | |
|---|---|
| **Planet/Star:** | Mercury |
| **Element:** | Air |
| **Colour vibration:** | Blue |
| **Gemstone:** | Emerald |
| | |
| **Top Strengths:** | Resourceful |
| | Multi-talented |
| | Good communicators |
| | Adaptable |
| | Charismatic |
| | |
| **Top Challenges:** | Addictive |
| | Melodramatic |
| | Intolerant |
| | Unfocused |
| | Changeable |

**Be Wary** – you can be quick-tempered, restless, impulsive and inconsistent.

**Guidance** – freedom and variety can be achieved in everyday life; it does not have to be 'the same old routine'.

**Career** – you are a natural storyteller, entertainer and counsellor. A freelancer or roles with face-to-face contact.

**Masculine** – active, creative, forward/aggressive, and cold.

## *Life Path – Number 5*

As a Life Path Number 5, you will have many of the following lessons to learn and work through in your lifetime.

### *The Life Lessons*

- You are to learn to be dynamic
- You are to learn to be full of energy
- You are to learn to be charming
- You are to learn to live for today
- You are to learn to be flexible and adaptable
- You are to learn to go with the flow of life
- You are to learn to be loyal in a relationship
- You are to learn to be smart and forward thinking
- You are to learn to enjoy going on an adventure
- You are to learn to be open to taking risks
- You are to learn to always be on the move and rarely sit still
- You are to learn to enjoy your freedom
- You are to learn to enjoy travelling and seeing new places
- You are to learn to be social
- You are to learn to make friends easily
- You are to learn to have your own mind
- You are to learn to be stimulated
- You are to learn to enjoy routine
- You are to learn not to be easily bored, if not engaged
- You are to learn not to be a poor judge of character
- You are to learn not to be ill-disciplined
- You are to learn not to lack focus and direction
- You are to learn not to be slow on the career ladder
- You are to learn not to procrastinate
- You are to learn not to be unreliable
- You are to learn not to succumb to drugs, drink, gambling…
- You are to learn not to be erratic

## *Expression – Number 5*

As an Expression Number 5, you chose to bring with you these talents and gifts to support your chosen Life Path Number.

- You are a natural adventurer
- You are destined to travel
- You are a thrill seeker
- You are multi-talented
- You are someone who enjoys having your freedom
- You are intelligent and quick-witted
- You are energetic
- You are an optimist
- You are a great communicator
- You are charming and charismatic
- You are often not in the present moment
- You are a people pleaser
- You are someone who may flitter between careers

## *Heart's Desire – Number 5*

As a Heart's Desire Number 5, you chose to bring with you these talents, gifts and passions to illuminate your life's purpose.

- You have a desire to be adventurous
- You have a desire to be full of energy and excitement
- You have a desire to be versatile and flexible
- You have a desire to be bright, witty and intelligent
- You have a desire to be inspirational
- You have a desire to travel
- You have a desire for change and variety
- You have a desire for anything new – people, places…etc.
- You have a desire to fulfil commitments
- You have a desire to be more patient
- You have a desire to be confident and charismatic
- You have a desire to be free from confinement or limitations
- You have a desire to be a risk-taker

## *Personality – Number 5*

As a Personality Number 5, you will have many of the following traits and focuses in your life.

- You are free-spirited
- You are adventurous
- You are a risk-taker
- You are confident
- You are a strong communicator
- You are optimistic
- You are charismatic
- You are intelligent
- You are an influencer
- You are a traveller
- You are flexible and adaptable
- You are approachable
- You are quick-witted

## *Birth Day – Number 5*

As a Birth Day Number 5, you will have many of the following traits and focuses in your life.

- You love variety and change
- You are a storyteller
- You are a traveller
- You are a natural adventurer
- You are a freedom seeker
- You are a pleasure to be around
- You are energetic and engaging
- You are inspiring at your best
- You are creative
- You are quick-witted and analytically minded
- You can lack patience
- You can overdo the good life
- You are a risk-taker

# Number 6

## The Counsellor – The Nurturer

Those connected with Number 6 are usually kind-natured and caring, always willing to listen and lend a hand whenever asked. The 6 is here to learn to be responsible without turning into a martyr.

| | |
|---|---|
| **Planet/Star:** | Venus |
| **Element:** | Earth |
| **Colour vibration:** | Indigo |
| **Gemstone:** | Diamond |
| | |
| **Top Strengths:** | Nurturing |
| | Supportive |
| | Sympathetic |
| | Loving |
| | Reliable |
| | |
| **Top Challenges:** | Bossy |
| | Critical |
| | Interfering |
| | Self-righteous |
| | Perfectionist |

**Be Wary** – you can be overbearing, a people pleaser, idealistic and have overly high expectations of yourself.

**Guidance** – live and let live, not everything needs to be controlled or monitored. Live in the moment. Enjoy the moment.

**Career** – positions using your empathy and kindness, such as a nurse, doctor, teacher, counsellor, home-worker or parent.

**Feminine** – passive, receptive, yielding and warm.

## *Life Path – Number 6*

As a Life Path Number 6, you will have many of the following lessons to learn and work through in your lifetime.

### *The Life Lessons*

- You are to learn to be the ultimate nurturer
- You are to learn to be truthful
- You are to learn to be a sympathetic and kind person
- You are to learn to be generous
- You are to learn to be dependable
- You are to learn to be an idealist
- You are to learn to be a perfectionist
- You are to learn to use your natural innocence
- You are to learn to set realistic targets for yourself
- You are to learn to have a paternal/maternal nature
- You are to learn to be head of the family
- You are to learn to revolve around home and family
- You are to learn to be a natural carer or caregiver
- You are to learn to lead by example
- You are to learn to always be willing to lend a hand
- You are to learn to use your tremendous wisdom
- You are to learn to have a strong sense of responsibility
- You are to learn to be a counsellor and teacher
- You are to learn to be a healer
- You are to learn to take on much responsibility
- You are to learn not to be self-critical
- You are to learn not to be self-sacrificing
- You are to learn not to be jealous
- You are to learn not to be a poor judge of character
- You are to learn not to be closed-minded
- You are to learn not to be stubborn
- You are to learn not to be vengeful or destructive

## *Expression – Number 6*

As an Expression Number 6, you chose to bring with you these talents and gifts to support your chosen Life Path Number.

- You are a natural nurturer
- You are loving and caring
- You are someone with a strong sense of duty
- You are intuitive
- You are responsible, reliable and trustworthy
- You are a counsellor – a great listener
- You are fair and just
- You are a giver
- You are someone who puts others ahead of yourself
- You are a calming influence in conflicts
- You are someone who can be overbearing
- You are someone who can be overprotective
- You are someone who can be patronising

## *Heart's Desire – Number 6*

As a Heart's Desire Number 6, you chose to bring with you these talents, gifts and passions to illuminate your life's purpose.

- You have a desire to be extremely loyal
- You have a desire to be caring
- You have a desire to enjoy family and friends around you
- You have a desire to help others
- You have a desire to be selfless
- You have a desire to be dependable
- You have a desire to be responsible
- You have a desire to be intuitive
- You have a desire to put others' needs ahead of your own
- You have a desire to be loving and nurturing
- You have a desire to be a person of principle and morals
- You have a desire to be wise
- You have a desire to be protective

## *Personality – Number 6*

As a Personality Number 6, you will have many of the following traits and focuses in your life.

- You are a nurturer
- You are sincere
- You are caring
- You are affectionate
- You are creative
- You are intuitive
- You are empathetic
- You are compassionate
- You are understanding
- You are wise
- You are supportive
- You are self-sacrificing
- You are righteous

## *Birth Day – Number 6*

As a Birth Day Number 6, you will have many of the following traits and focuses in your life.

- You love home and family
- You are a perfectionist
- You enjoy traditions and family values
- You are responsible
- You are a nurturer
- You love helping others
- You are artistic
- You enjoy peace and harmony
- You are naturally caring
- You are a strong mediator
- You have the ability to be a healer
- You are intuitive
- You are compassionate and understanding

# Number 7

## The Philosopher – The Analyst

Anyone connected with the Number 7 is usually analytical by nature and can often be something of an introvert. They often care less about what others think of them and care more about what they are focused on. The 7 is here to learn how to trust in a Divine connection while losing the need to overthink.

| | |
|---|---|
| **Planet/Star:** | Neptune |
| **Element:** | Water |
| **Colour vibration:** | Violet |
| **Gemstone:** | Cat's eye |
| | |
| **Top Strengths:** | Intellectual |
| | Technically-orientated |
| | Investigative |
| | Intuitive |
| | Analytical |
| | |
| **Top Challenges:** | Intolerant |
| | Secretive |
| | Pessimistic |
| | Cynical |
| | Suspicious |

**Be Wary** – you can close yourself off emotionally and avoid all emotions. You can be selfish, opinionated and a loner.

**Guidance** – being alone is not the same as loneliness, trust your intuition and connect with more likeminded people.

**Career** – a professor, philosopher or guru within science or academia. Working alone is where you are happiest.

**Masculine** – active, creative, forward/aggressive, and cold.

## *Life Path – Number 7*

As a Life Path Number 7, you will have many of the following lessons to learn and work through in your lifetime.

### *The Life Lessons*

- You are to learn to be a peaceful person
- You are to learn to be a harmonious person
- You are to learn to be a deep thinker
- You are to learn to be an intellectual
- You are to learn to be philosophical
- You are to learn to be intuitive
- You are to learn to think about worlds further than Earth
- You are to learn to have a great ability to read people
- You are to learn to be a good judge of character
- You are to learn to be socially outgoing
- You are to learn to have a core of trusted friends/ colleagues
- You are to learn to be comfortable on your own
- You are to learn to be intuitive and use your gut instincts
- You are to learn to manage major mood shifts
- You are to learn to find balance in your life
- You are to learn to draw your own conclusions rather than believing others
- You are to learn not to be overly motivated by money
- You are to learn not to be insecure or have insecurities
- You are to learn not to be cynical
- You are to learn not to be defensive and guarded
- You are to learn not to be cold-hearted and tactless
- You are to learn not to lack empathy
- You are to learn not to lack contact with the world
- You are to learn not to be selfish
- You are to learn not to give up too easily

## *Expression – Number 7*

As an Expression Number 7, you chose to bring with you these talents and gifts to support your chosen Life Path Number.

- You are very intuitive
- You are intelligent
- You are philosophical and a deep thinker
- You are someone who seeks truth and understanding
- You are someone who enjoys your personal space
- You are introverted
- You are motivated by understanding more
- You are analytically minded
- You are someone who has a need to find answers
- You are very self-protecting
- You are someone who can be mistrustful
- You are someone who does not share the full truth
- You are someone who can lack empathy

## *Heart's Desire – Number 7*

As a Heart's Desire Number 7, you chose to bring with you these talents, gifts and passions to illuminate your life's purpose.

- You have a desire to be analytical
- You have a desire to be studious
- You have a desire to be a deep thinker
- You have a desire to be independent
- You have a desire to focus on the now and waste little time
- You have a desire to be a perfectionist
- You have a desire to be philosophical
- You have a desire for personal space
- You have a desire to be driven by a need for answers
- You have a desire to be a natural researcher
- You have a desire not to be withdrawn
- You have a desire not to be rigid and inflexible
- You have a desire not to be secretive

## *Personality – Number 7*

As a Personality Number 7, you will have many of the following traits and focuses in your life.

- You are a deep thinker
- You are analytical
- You are introverted
- You are intuitive
- You are quick-witted
- You are mysterious
- You are wise
- You are inspiring
- You are spiritual or religious
- You are outgoing
- You are intriguing
- You are intelligent
- You are secretive

## *Birth Day – Number 7*

As a Birth Day Number 7, you will have many of the following traits and focuses in your life.

- You love time to yourself
- You enjoy peace and quiet
- You enjoy nature and all that it holds
- You have a highly developed mind
- You enjoy metaphysical studies
- You are studious and enjoy research
- You are intelligent
- You have a keen intuition
- You prefer to work alone
- You are sensitive and feel deeply
- You have trouble opening up to people
- You can be secretive
- You can be stubborn, cynical and cold

# Number 8

## The Visionary – The Business Leader

In China, 8 is an incredibly lucky number. This number is often a symbol of abundance and prosperity. Those associated with the number 8 are usually surrounded by success in their lives. The 8 is here to learn how to chase opportunities to serve, rather than chase opportunities to make money.

| | |
|---|---|
| **Planet/Star:** | Saturn |
| **Element:** | Earth |
| **Colour vibration:** | Rose |
| **Gemstone:** | Blue Sapphire |
| | |
| **Top Strengths:** | Organised |
| | Self-motivated |
| | Driven |
| | Strong |
| | Hard working |
| | |
| **Top Challenges:** | Domineering |
| | Poverty-conscious |
| | Superficial |
| | Intimidating |
| | Manipulative |

**Be Wary** – you can be stubborn, ruthless and a workaholic.
**Guidance** – understand that power and money can be used for the greater good, not only for your own purposes.
**Career** – you are a natural leader and a strong businessperson. Money and power are what you strive for. A position as CEO or entrepreneur in banking, finance or commerce.
**Feminine** – passive, receptive, yielding and warm.

## *Life Path – Number 8*

As a Life Path Number 8, you will have many of the following lessons to learn and work through in your lifetime.

### *The Life Lessons*

- You are to learn to be a natural leader
- You are to learn to be a great manager
- You are to learn to have a great understanding of business
- You are to learn to be energetic
- You are to learn to be driven and ambitious
- You are to learn to be focused and determined
- You are to learn to be naturally organised
- You are to learn to be a realist and visionary
- You are to learn to have a positive mindset
- You are to learn to believe that anything is possible
- You are to learn to be an inspiration to others
- You are to learn to look longer-term in the future
- You are to learn to have the Midas touch (golden touch)
- You are to learn to focus on business and finance
- You are to learn to be a doer
- You are to learn to have a positive nature and personality
- You are to learn to be a problem solver
- You are to learn to be generous
- You are to learn not to use wealth to the detriment of others
- You are to learn not to be materialistic
- You are to learn not to be intolerant of others
- You are to learn not to be risk averse
- You are to learn not to give up
- You are to learn not to take 'no' for an answer
- You are to learn not to feel personally unsatisfied
- You are to learn not to lack confidence in yourself

## *Expression – Number 8*

As an Expression Number 8, you chose to bring with you these talents and gifts to support your chosen Life Path Number.

- You are very competitive
- You are hard working
- You are ambitious
- You are a visionary
- You are a leader, manager and team leader
- You are efficient and effective
- You are driven to succeed in your chosen field
- You are organised and well planned
- You are a fantastic judge of character
- You are someone who balances success and cares for others
- You are loyal to those that are loyal to you
- You are someone who rewards hard work and results
- You are self-confident

## *Heart's Desire – Number 8*

As a Heart's Desire Number 8, you chose to bring with you these talents, gifts and passions to illuminate your life's purpose.

- You have a desire for success and power
- You have a desire to be analytical
- You have a desire to be a great judge of character
- You have a desire for results and achievement
- You have a desire to achieve your goals
- You have a desire to be a visionary
- You have a desire to work well in a team
- You have a desire to inspire and develop others
- You have a desire to be calm in times of stress or crisis
- You have a desire not to be self-centred
- You have a desire not to be emotionally repressed
- You have a desire not to be overly materialistic
- You have a desire not to be domineering

## *Personality – Number 8*

As a Personality Number 8, you will have many of the following traits and focuses in your life.

- You are a visionary
- You are a leader
- You are ambitious
- You are confident
- You are strong
- You are goal-orientated
- You are results focused
- You are successful
- You are a planner
- You are organised
- You are passionate
- You are a positive person
- You are overpowering

## *Birth Day – Number 8*

As a Birth Day Number 8, you will have many of the following traits and focuses in your life.

- You like to take charge and lead
- You are focused on quality over quantity
- You are an achiever
- You are a strategist and planner
- You are highly competitive
- You have a need to win at all costs
- You are destined for high positions of power
- You are efficient
- You are results-driven
- You are a good judge of character
- You have an intolerance for weakness
- You can be domineering or bossy
- You are a positive person

# Number 9

## The Philanthropist – The Humanitarian

Those with the number 9 in their path are associated with peace, selflessness and empathy. The 9 is here to learn how to be a healer, while eradicating the need to be a hero in favour of teaching others how to help themselves.

| | |
|---|---|
| **Planet/Star:** | Mars |
| **Element:** | Fire |
| **Colour vibration:** | Gold |
| **Gemstone:** | Coral |
| | |
| **Top Strengths:** | Compassionate |
| | Generous |
| | Passionate |
| | Broad-minded |
| | Sympathetic |
| | |
| **Top Challenges:** | Unforgiving |
| | Revengeful |
| | Defensive |
| | Melodramatic |
| | Aggressive |

**Be Wary** – you can find it hard to let go, you can be misunderstood, isolated and overly giving.

**Guidance** – forgive and forget, this will release you from old wounds. Live in the present moment.

**Career** – you are a natural teacher and counsellor, a career assisting others will serve you well.

**Masculine** – active, creative, forward/aggressive, and cold.

## *Life Path – Number 9*

As a Life Path Number 9, you will have many of the following lessons to learn and work through in your lifetime.

## *The Life Lessons*

- You are to learn to be honourable
- You are to learn to be trustworthy and loyal
- You are to learn to be compassionate
- You are to learn to care about those less fortunate
- You are to learn to have a desire to help mankind
- You are to learn to be able to make new friends easily
- You are to learn to have an open and magnetic personality
- You are to learn to have a positive and upbeat personality
- You are to learn to be at the top in your chosen field
- You are to learn to be sensitive and feel emotions greatly
- You are to learn to have a deep understanding of life
- You are to learn to be drawn to the arts or literary fields
- You are to learn to have humanitarian inclinations
- You are to learn to make the world a better place
- You are to learn to be creative
- You are to learn to be charismatic and have magnetism
- You are to learn to be a leader
- You are to learn to achieve great wealth
- You are to learn to write, act, dance, design or paint
- You are to learn to care about the greater good
- You are to learn not to hide your emotions
- You are to learn not to be a demanding partner
- You are to learn not to be cold and defensive
- You are to learn not to be egotistical
- You are to learn not to be cruel and malicious
- You are to learn not to be immoral
- You are to learn not to temperamental

## *Expression – Number 9*

As an Expression Number 9, you chose to bring with you these talents and gifts to support your chosen Life Path Number.

- You are a natural humanitarian
- You are charismatic
- You are someone who inspires others to achieve for more
- You are someone who has a need for love and admiration
- You are compassionate
- You are generous
- You are nurturing
- You are someone who focuses on bettering mankind
- You are absent of prejudice
- You are artistic and creative
- You are selfless for the greater good
- You are not a strong judge of character
- You are someone who looks at the bigger picture

## *Heart's Desire – Number 9*

As a Heart's Desire Number 9, you chose to bring with you these talents, gifts and passions to illuminate your life's purpose.

- You have a desire to be a philanthropist
- You have a desire to serve mankind
- You have a desire to make the world a better place
- You have a desire to play your part for humanity
- You have a desire to be a perfectionist
- You have a desire to help as many people as you can
- You have a desire to have an idealistic nature
- You have a desire to be highly intuitive
- You have a desire to be selfless
- You have a desire to help people develop in their lives
- You have a desire to be generous and nurturing
- You have a desire not to be idealistic with your goals
- You have a desire not to be arrogant

## *Personality – Number 9*

As a Personality Number 9, you will have many of the following traits and focuses in your life.

- You are a humanitarian
- You are a philanthropist
- You are empathetic
- You are generous
- You are compassionate
- You are loyal
- You are nurturing
- You are creative
- You are charismatic
- You are noble and dignified
- You are intolerant
- You are arrogant
- You are self-serving

## *Birth Day – Number 9*

As a Birth Day Number 9, you will have many of the following traits and focuses in your life.

- You love to help others
- You are a problem solver
- You are a giver
- You love the arts and music
- You are a visionary
- You are an idealist
- You are a compassionate person at heart
- You are sociable
- You are charismatic
- You are open-minded
- You are creative
- You are naturally 'lucky'
- You are loyal

# The Master Numbers 11, 22 And 33

In Numerology there are additional numbers that are said to hold significant meaning and importance; these numbers are 11, 22 and 33 (44 is possible although unlikely to arise in a numerology chart). These three Master Numbers are never reduced within numerology calculations due to their unique significance and are believed to be at a higher vibration than their reduced number (11/2, 22/4 and 33/6).

It is believed by many modern numerologists that those with a Master Number of 11, 22 or 33 as their Life Path, Expression Number or Heart's Desire Number are old souls that have been incarnated many times and have much spiritual knowledge. Master Numbers can carry with them a weight of expectation and workload in the physical form, therefore it is understood that each person with a Master Number as a core number has the decision on whether they use this special knowledge in their lives and assist in raising awareness of the collective consciousness of Earth, and all those living within.

Master Numbers are not the masters of anything. Those with a Master Number in their chart are here to 'master' the double vibration associated with the duplicated number to the left of the slash. For example, a person with an 11/2 Life Path would have to 'master' the double vibration of the number 1. Many people are disappointed when they find out they are not Master Numbers. They feel there is some notoriety associated with being a Master Number, which is simply not the case.

Having a Master Number in your path is also believed to be similar to taking a Master's Degree of life. One that is likely to have many challenges and obstacles that will push you to the point of breaking; however, you are always able to overcome and succeed in whatever is put in front of you. Any experience or situation that life throws at you is there for a purpose, it is there for you to learn from the lesson/s in the situation, understand them and move on. There will never be a situation put in front of you that you will not be able to manage. You will always have the tools and talent available to you.

Master 11s are a complex group of individuals; 11s rarely feel good enough within themselves. They are always looking for the next best thing and can often sabotage their own efforts. 11s need to understand that they are not here to improve on something that someone else has done before them. 11s are here to create something entirely of their own doing. They need to do something that no one has ever done before. They need to bring originality rather than duplication.

Master 22s feel the need to be the master builders of something; however, similar to that of the 11s they often do not succeed because they have no idea what they are intended to build. The clue lies in the fact that 22s fail to realise that they are not here to do this by themselves. The double 2 energy emphasises the need for partnership. They need to align themselves with others with a similar mindset who buy into their vision and will assist them in building something that will benefit humanity.

Master 33s are somewhat rare. They are here to work through the challenges related to their need for perfectionism. They often suffer from extreme self-doubt, which can only be remedied once they choose to honour the moment while appreciating the perfection that exists in all things. The Master 33s are the most sensitive of all the Master Numbers. They (33/6s) are balancing their need for creative emotional expression related to the vibration of the double 3, with the desire for perfection that comes from the 6. Once they accept that perfection exists in all things, they soon accept the perfection that exists within themselves.

# Master Number 11

## The Master Healer (connected with No. 2)

Number 11 is a balance between numbers 1 and 2, which is in itself conflicted as 1 and 2 are complete opposites. Number 11 is said to be the most intuitive of all numbers and represents illumination, intuition, truth, knowledge and inspiration.

**Top Strengths:**
Intuitive
Broad-minded
Inspirational
Uplifting
Peacemaker

**Top Challenges:**
Insecure
Dishonest
Intense
Delusional
Hypersensitive

**Be Wary** – you can be constantly tested on your journey from life's lessons. You often seek the approval of others.
**Guidance** – the only person you need to listen to is your own intuition, this is fulfilment enough.
**Career** – as a natural leader, teacher and guide, you need to follow your own intuition. Forge your own path and lead from the front.
**Feminine and Masculine** – passive, receptive, yielding, warm, active, creative, forward/aggressive and cold.

## *Life Path – Master Number 11*

As a Life Path Number 11, you will have many of the following lessons to learn and work through in your lifetime.

### *The Life Lessons*

- You are to learn to be the Master Healer
- You are to learn to be the 'Wounded Healer'
- You are to learn to be a natural teacher
- You are to learn to be instinctive
- You are to learn to be highly intuitive
- You are to learn to be energetic
- You are to learn to be passionate
- You are to learn to be empathetic
- You are to learn to uplift and inspire
- You are to learn to be creative
- You are to learn to be a great leader
- You are to learn to be a wonderful listener
- You are to learn to be calm in difficult situations
- You are to learn to be old beyond your years
- You are to learn to be described as an old soul
- You are to learn to breathe life into every situation
- You are to learn to illuminate with your message
- You are to learn to know without rationality
- You are to learn to enjoy and promote harmony
- You are to learn to achieve something monumental
- You are to learn to promote peace, healing and spiritual awareness
- You are to learn to have a strong connection with your subconscious
- You are to learn not to be overly sensitive
- You are to learn not to be anxious and fearful
- You are to learn not to be shy and withdrawn

## *Expression – Master Number 11*

As an Expression Number 11, you chose to bring with you these talents and gifts to support your chosen Life Path Number.

- You are a natural psychic
- You are very intelligent
- You are logical and creative
- You are a hard worker
- You are a natural teacher and mentor
- You are kind and passionate
- You are extremely sensitive
- You are aware of higher levels of consciousness
- You are creative and inspiring
- You are spiritual
- You are an attentive listener
- You are someone who can be anxious and fearful
- You are someone who can be shy and withdrawn

## *Heart's Desire – Master Number 11*

As a Heart's Desire Number 11, you chose to bring with you these talents, gifts and passions to illuminate your life's purpose.

- You have a desire to be the Master Healer
- You have a desire to be a spiritual seeker and visionary
- You have a desire to be a messenger for the metaphysical
- You have a desire to help others in finding their potential
- You have a desire to be an old soul and have wisdom
- You have a desire to understand the significance of life
- You have a desire to use your experiences to assist others
- You have a desire to have a great deal of empathy for others
- You have a desire to be creative and philosophical
- You have a desire to be a natural peacemaker and seek enlightenment
- You have a desire to heal the world and make it a better place

## *Personality – Master Number 11*

As a Personality Number 11, you will have many of the following traits and focuses in your life.

- You are inspirational
- You are spiritual
- You are intuitive
- You are creative
- You are kind
- You are imaginative
- You are insightful
- You are a great listener
- You are shy and introverted
- You are someone who enjoys the finer things in life
- You are to make others feel important, loved and wanted
- You are someone who hates conflict and disharmony
- You are someone who can lack self-confidence

## *Birth Day – Master Number 11*

As a Birth Day Number 11, you will have many of the following traits and focuses in your life.

- You love to mentor and help others
- You have a strong interest in the metaphysical
- You are a teacher and messenger
- You are a facilitator
- You are highly intuitive and insightful
- You are very in-tune with your inner-self
- You are a natural healer
- You are an inspirational figure for others
- You are able to help others reach their full potential
- You are determined and focused when a goal is set
- You are a great and compassionate leader
- You are very sensitive and can be highly emotional
- You are imaginative

# Master Number 22

## The Master Builder (connected with No. 4)

Master Number 22 is said to be the most powerful of all numbers and is called the Master Builder. The Master Number 22 has the ability to turn the most ambitious of dreams into reality when it is supported by other core numbers in the chart.

| | |
|---|---|
| **Top Strengths:** | Visionary |
| | Forward thinking |
| | Dedicated |
| | Focused |
| | Idealistic |
| | |
| **Top Challenges:** | Inflexible |
| | Workaholic |
| | Stubborn |
| | Controlling |
| | Perfectionist |

**Be Wary** – do not take on too much responsibility, especially when you are not being valued by those you are helping. You can be insecure and bossy.

**Guidance** – the trials, tests and tribulations that arise throughout life are all there for you to reach your greatest potential. They are there for your greater good.

**Career** – you are a natural teacher, leader, humanitarian and philanthropist.

**Feminine** – passive, receptive, yielding and warm.

## *Life Path – Master Number 22*

As a Life Path Number 22, you will have many of the following lessons to learn and work through in your lifetime.

### *The Life Lessons*

- You are to learn to be the Master Builder
- You are to learn to be a doer and a go-getter
- You are to learn to turn dreams into reality
- You are to learn to be a success
- You are to learn to be psychic
- You are to learn to be a forward thinker
- You are to learn to be trustworthy and honourable
- You are to learn to be grounded by nature
- You are to learn to enjoy your freedom and independence
- You are to learn to be ambitious and disciplined
- You are to learn to be a strong leader
- You are to learn to be a big thinker
- You are to learn to be a strong communicator
- You are to learn to be very confident
- You are to learn to be willing to take risks
- You are to learn to be intuitive
- You are to learn to work hard to fulfil your potential
- You are to learn to be materially successful
- You are to learn to be honest
- You are to learn to be hard working
- You are to learn to take one step at a time
- You are to learn to have patience
- You are to learn to have perseverance
- You are to learn to spend time understanding yourself
- You are to learn not to lack self-confidence
- You are to learn not to be highly sensitive
- You are to learn not to be sensitive to negative energies

## *Expression – Master Number 22*

As an Expression Number 22, you chose to bring with you these talents and gifts to support your chosen Life Path Number.

- You are naturally psychic
- You are the Master Builder
- You are a visionary
- You are a strong leader
- You are organised and diligent
- You are highly intuitive
- You are very confident
- You are someone who can make a difference to the world
- You are someone who can accomplish much greatness
- You are someone who has no limits to your capability
- You are aware of the big picture and see more than others
- You are someone who can be too focused on material gains
- You are sensitive to the energies of those around you

## *Heart's Desire – Master Number 22*

As a Heart's Desire Number 22, you chose to bring with you these talents, gifts and passions to illuminate your life's purpose.

- You have a desire to be innovative and creative
- You have a desire to be intelligent
- You have a desire to be an overachiever
- You have a desire to better mankind
- You have a desire to be confident
- You have a desire to be sensible and pragmatic
- You have a desire to leave a lasting legacy
- You have a desire to make dreams happen
- You have a desire to accept much responsibility in life
- You have a desire to be a leader of people
- You have a desire to reach great heights in this lifetime
- You have a desire to learn in life before progressing
- You have a desire not to be highly sensitive

## *Personality – Master Number 22*

As a Personality Number 22, you will have many of the following traits and focuses in your life.

- You are a Master Builder
- You are a forward thinker and visionary
- You are a creator and designer
- You are inspirational
- You are very confident in yourself
- You are trustworthy and honourable
- You are highly intelligent and hard working
- You are very sensitive
- You are extremely creative
- You are someone who can turn your ambitions into reality
- You are dependable and reliable
- You are a great leader
- You are someone who can have self-doubt

## *Birth Day – Master Number 22*

As a Birth Day Number 22, you will have many of the following traits and focuses in your life.

- You are a Master Builder
- You are extremely capable
- You are a great leader
- You are here to assist mankind and humanity
- You are a visionary and idealistic
- You are detail-orientated
- You have huge potential for success
- You are honest and sensitive
- You are very smart and creative
- You are destined for great things
- You can achieve your heart's desires
- You can have a fear of failure
- You can be overly confident and aggressive

# Master Number 33

## The Master Nurturer/Teacher (connected with No. 6)

Master Number 33 is one of the rarest numbers within numerology as only a small percentage of people have a birthdate that reduces down to the Master Number 33. The Master Number 33 is said to be one of the most influential and important numbers, linking with the number 6. Master Number 33 is often called the Master Teacher and is the most spiritually evolved of all numbers.

| | |
|---|---|
| **Top Strengths:** | Creative |
| | Healing |
| | Compassionate |
| | Loving |
| | Nurturing |
| | |
| **Top Challenges:** | Perfectionist |
| | Overachieving |
| | Critical |
| | Self-righteous |
| | Self-critical |

**Be Wary** – you can neglect yourself, be a perfectionist and lack self-appreciation. You have a need for balance.
**Guidance** – you are all you need to be, right this very moment. Enjoy being you.
**Career** – you are a natural nurturer, caregiver, teacher, counsellor, charitable worker, humanitarian or homemaker.
**Feminine and Masculine** – passive, receptive, yielding, warm, active, creative, forward/aggressive, and cold.

## *Life Path – Master Number 33*

As a Life Path Number 33, you will have many of the following lessons to learn and work through in your lifetime.

## *The Life Lessons*

- You are to learn to be the Master Teacher
- You are to learn to be a humanitarian
- You are to learn to be highly knowledgeable
- You are to learn to be practical
- You are to learn to prefer facts over fiction
- You are to learn to be extremely creative
- You are to learn to use your abilities to better others
- You are to learn to have a natural concern for the planet
- You are to learn to want to save everyone
- You are to learn to be very intuitive
- You are to learn to be sensitive
- You are to learn to be naturally nurturing
- You are to learn to be responsible and reliable
- You are to learn to appreciate and enjoy the arts
- You are to learn to be an expressive person
- You are to learn to be loving and caring
- You are to learn to be devoted to your specific cause
- You are to learn to be a healer
- You are to learn not to be impulsive
- You are to learn not to be hyperactive
- You are to learn not to be too much of a perfectionist
- You are to learn not to be hypersensitive
- You are to learn not to take on too much responsibility
- You are to learn not to be insecure
- You are to learn not to seek approval from others
- You are to learn not to have high expectations of yourself
- You are to learn not to self-sacrifice

## *Expression – Master Number 33*

As an Expression Number 33, you chose to bring with you these talents and gifts to support your chosen Life Path Number.

- You are the Master Nurturer
- You are a teacher, mentor and coach
- You are spiritual
- You are someone with extremely high expectations
- You are loving and caring
- You are very intuitive
- You are someone who lives in peace and harmony
- You are self-sacrificing
- You are action-orientated
- You are a healer and a humanitarian
- You are empathetic and creative
- You are someone with a need to help the world
- You are giving of yourself to good causes and help others

## *Heart's Desire – Master Number 33*

As a Heart's Desire Number 33, you chose to bring with you these talents, gifts and passions to illuminate your life's purpose.

- You have a desire to be a Master Teacher
- You have a desire to be creative and practical
- You have a desire to be a healer
- You have a desire to progress and heal mankind
- You have a desire to assist the betterment of the planet
- You have a desire to be a humanitarian
- You have a desire to be intuitive and idealistic
- You have a desire to be driven by facts and not fiction
- You have a desire to be an achiever
- You have a desire to be a leader, mentor and coach
- You have a desire to be thoughtful
- You have a desire to take action
- You have a desire not to rest on your laurels

## *Personality – Master Number 33*

As a Personality Number 33, you will have many of the following traits and focuses in your life.

- You are a Master Teacher
- You are someone who desires to leave a lasting legacy
- You are sensitive and loving
- You are giving of yourself to others and good causes
- You are thoughtful and practical
- You are highly intelligent and very creative
- You are very intuitive
- You are a humanitarian and idealistic
- You are someone who has high expectations of yourself
- You are always on the go
- You are someone who checks facts before giving an opinion
- You are sensible and reliable
- You are someone who has a need to learn patience

## *Birth Day – Master Number 33*

As there is no birth date 33, we take the relationship between the number 33 and the number 6 (3+3=6) to assist us with the Birth Day number for 33.

- You love home and family
- You are a perfectionist
- You enjoy traditions and family values
- You are responsible
- You are a nurturer
- You love helping others
- You are artistic
- You enjoy peace and harmony
- You are naturally caring
- You are a strong mediator
- You have the ability to be a healer
- You can be arrogant

# Ann Perry

### International Numerologist

This chapter has been edited with the assistance of Ann Perry, international numerologist.

Ann Perry is a professional numerologist who specialises in numerology workshops, readings and intensive personalised courses. Her purpose is to help you to discover yours.

If you feel connected and empowered by the workings of numerology, contact Ann for a detailed personalised reading.

Use this reference when making contact:
**THE HOLISTIC GUIDE**

Website: www.annperrynumerologist.com

# Numbers: The Universal Language

*Nature is written in mathematical language.*
Galileo Galilei

# The Universe And The Number Messages Within

This chapter has been edited with the assistance of Ann Perry, international numerologist.

As has been said numerous times thus far in this book, the world and everything within it is connected and is made up of numbers, equations and mathematics. Whether this is the individual fingerprints on your hand, your DNA or the lines on a bark through a tree, everything in its own right has a unique code, and a number code at that. Everything we can see, feel and touch has a number code. Numbers are truly the language of the universe, and we are able to receive these Universal Number messages.

You may have seen or come across reoccurring numbers in your everyday life. These numbers or messages are often called G-d Numbers, Angel Numbers or Universal Numbers. These Universal Number messages are all around us on a continual basis and are directed towards us to offer guidance, a warning, comfort or something more. Thousands and thousands of people from all over the world have reported noticing specific number sequences on watches, clocks, hotel rooms, telephone numbers, advertising billboards, number plates, views of a news story, number of comments, the time of a message, mobile telephones, computers etc. If you have ever noticed the same numbers reoccurring in your life, these are universal messages of guidance and direction for you.

From my own personal experience, I have always been drawn to numbers and the power of the number. That said, it was around the age of 34 that I started noticing specific number patterns everywhere, from seeing the same time on my watch, clock, phone and computer, to having the same number office, hotel rooms and advertising boards. Not only this, when a number message is in front of me, I feel a specific and energetic pull (almost like a light switch) for me to look at the time or number code (wherever this may be). This is another link to the energy system of the chakras and the energy transducers (pineal gland). The first number codes that most people see are 111 or 1111 and 333. These numbers were prevalent around me for some time. I would even show others, including my wife, when they continuously appeared and reappeared.

Now some years later, and more knowledgeable on the subject, I have been able to understand the Universal Number's guidance and direction, with the help of well-renowned Universal Number specialists, such as Joanne Walmsley and Kyle Gray. With numbers being the language of the universe, it is up to us to be in-tune, present and awake enough to take notice so that we can understand the messages, guidance and communications we are being offered by the universe. These are messages of the universe, and they speak to us all the time. We only have to attune ourselves and take note of the messages as they arise.

According to respected authors, therapists, numerologists and spiritualists at all corners of the world, these universal messages are occurring as a new Spiritual Awareness is taking place and gaining momentum on our planet. As a race of people, we are evolving on a spiritual level, with the Universal Number sequences being 'messages' from a higher vibration or source.

The universe hopes that we will be aware enough and acknowledge that we are seeing the same number sequences, time and time again. It wants us to notice what the number message is and then look further into the meanings of the messages to receive its fullest guidance.

## The Numbers: The Hidden Meanings

In the section below, each number has been broken down into what the number represents and is associated with individually within the Universal Number messages.

### *What Does It All Mean?*

NUMBER 0

Zero is associated with emptiness, completeness and the whole. Zero represents that you are on the right path.

NUMBER 1

One is connected with change, a new beginning and overcoming negativity.

NUMBER 2

Two represents peace, balance and harmony. It is also associated with relationships (business and personal).

NUMBER 3

Three is connected with wisdom, connection and chasing your dreams.

NUMBER 4

Four represents routine, stability and patience.

NUMBER 5

Five is associated with change and progress.

NUMBER 6

Six is connected to your inner-self and keeping a balance with the material world.

**NUMBER 7**       Seven represents positivity, personal achievement and universal awakening.

**NUMBER 8**       Eight connects to success, abundance and prosperity.

**NUMBER 9**       Nine is linked to compassion and empathy.

# The Universal Number Messages

Within this chapter we focus on the major aspects of the number messages within each sequence, with the assistance of Joanne Walmsley (spiritualist), Ann Perry (numerologist), Doreen Virtue (doctor of psychology) and Kyle Gray (spiritualist).

Numbers hold messages and the combination of these numbers can be decoded. While it is a great place to start, and very useful, the interpretation of those messages needs to come from within and not explicitly from external sources. There are many wonderful numerologists and numerology guides; however, it is always important to search within ourselves for what messages connect and resonate with us. Only you know the true value of the message in the repeated number sequences. It is really up to you to decipher the message. The numbers are clues that can help.

Each number message has deeper meaning, and it is recommended that you research further, should a message strike a chord with you.

## Reoccurring Triple And Quadruple Numbers

All the number sequences below relate to those triple and quadruple numbers that are regularly seen in everyday life on a reoccurring basis.

### *Number 000 or 0000*

This number often indicates a new start or the beginning of a journey. This is a message telling you that now is a great time to start your new adventure. Number 0000 is associated with financial stability and life progression.

### *Number 111 or 1111*

Number 111 is connected with your thoughts and dreams turning to reality. Let go of any fears and doubts you have, focus only on your goals. Believe that everything is possible and achievable. Only think positively.

### *Number 222 or 2222*

Numbers 222 and 2222 are linked to harmony, peace and balance. This number encourages you to take a balanced and harmonious view in every part of your life. 222 also brings with it a positive message of work well done and achievement. Keep up the good work and have faith!

### *Number 333 or 3333*

Number 333 is connected with the Ascended Masters (Jesus, Moses, Buddha, Shiva etc.). This number brings with it a message of love, support, guidance and protection. Your prayers have been heard and you are being cared for. Trust in the universe, and believe.

## Number 444 or 4444

This brings a message of positivity, encouragement and patience. Everything happens in its own right time. Numbers 444 and 4444 are connected to work, practicality and connection. You are on the right path; keep doing what you are doing and in time you will see the fruits of your labour. Do not give up!

## Number 555 or 5555

Number 555 indicates widescale change across many fronts in your life. This is a message to ask you to remain positive and focused on your goals during this time of change. Remain positive and keep the faith! Remember that anything that is taken from you will be replaced with better and will serve you more positively on your journey.

## Number 666 or 6666

This is a number sequence that often conveys negative imagery. The number 6666 is linked to a negative focus on the material world, caring too much about money and not enough about yourself and family life. This is a message to bring balance into your life and focus on other areas.

## Number 777 or 7777

Number 777 brings a message from the universe that you are on the correct path in all areas of your life. Continue to stay balanced and focused to positively progress on this path. Number 777 also reminds you that in this lifetime you are here to universally evolve. Embrace your unique talents and fully express yourself for the service and benefit of others.

## *Number 888 or 8888*

This is a message of financial gain, support and reward from the universe. Numbers 888 and 8888 bring an encouraging message of money flowing in your direction. Ensure that you create a solid foundation for you and your family; this will cement your future prosperity. Number 888 reminds you of your integrity and being true to who you are.

## *Number 999 or 9999*

Number 999 is often associated with an ending or closing of a chapter. A situation or phase of your life is coming to a close or will soon end naturally. This number brings you a message of progression and a call to action. Now is the time for you to get to work on your life's purpose. Trust that all you require will be provided by the universe.

## Mirror Time Numbers

All the number sequences below relate to those mirror image numbers that are regularly seen in a 24-hour clock on a reoccurring basis. The following number sequences take the energy of more than one number to create a balanced message from each characteristic within the numbers.

### Number 101, 0101 or 1010

Number 101 is connected with personal development, awakening and enlightenment. The universe is sending a message that this is the time to focus your attention on your soul's desire and inner-calling. Take this as a call to action, step forward positively and have faith that you will find personal success and achievement.

### Number 202, 0202 or 2020

The universe brings a positive message, your thoughts and dreams can turn into reality. Keep a positive mindset and have clear and defined goals. With balance, harmony and belief, miracles can truly happen in your life.

### Number 303, 0303 or 3030

Number 303 is connected to the Ascended Masters and new beginnings. You are being guided to follow your intuition and start a new venture or project you are thinking about. Now is your time to act. Have faith that you will be guided and protected by the universe and all within it. Your prayers have been answered.

### Number 404, 0404 or 4040

Number 404 is a message that your hard work and dedication have not gone unnoticed. By serving your soul's purpose you are achieving in all you do. Continue to progress forward with passion, confidence and enthusiasm. Know that you are surrounded and protected by the Universal Energies.

### Number 505, 0505 or 5050

The number 5 is associated with change, and when combined with the 0s' vibration suggests of breaking free, moving in a new direction and seeking new horizons. Universal Number 505 brings an important message of needed and necessary change in your life. This is the time to break free from anything holding you back and take a chance.

### Number 606, 0606 or 6060

This is a message that asks you to look into the spiritual and humanitarian world, rather than the material world. You are too focused on financial gain and material items. This is a message to refocus your sights on what is genuinely important. Believe that you are able to make these changes for the betterment and benefit of your life.

### Number 707, 0707 or 7070

Universal Number 707 is a message of praise, pride and a pat on the back. Your hard work and dedication to yourself and others in your life has been recognised and commended by the Universal Energies. You are being asked to continue your positive and inspirational work. Thank you!

## Number 808, 0808 or 8080

The number 8 is often connected with abundance, here is no different. The universe tells you of abundant opportunities, changes and ideas. Guidance and help are available to you. You must be aware and alert to the opportunities in front of you, these are the answers to your prayers. You need to be ready to receive the gifts you are being offered.

## Number 909, 0909 or 9090

Universal Number 909 comes with a message of change or progression. While there are changes happening in your life, have faith and belief that these changes will ultimately work out for the best and will be a blessing in disguise. Let go, and have faith!

## Number 1212 or 2121

With a combination of both numbers 1 and 2, this number sequence brings a message of faith, belief and new directions. Believe that you have the ability to step outside of your comfort zone and begin a new venture or head in a new direction. Trust in yourself and your intuition, listen to the messages from your inner core and release all fears.

## Number 1313 or 3131

Number 1313 is a sign from the universe that you are being guided and directed by the Universal Energies to ensure you are able to walk your chosen path with a positive and optimistic mindset. Be ready to experience new opportunities to expand your horizons and express yourself fully. Use your unique talents to create joy and happiness in your life and the lives of others.

## *Number 1414 or 4141*

This number is connected to having a continued positive mindset and releasing your worries and concerns. Number 1414 or 4141 is a universal message that your energies are being positively elevated to guide you along your path. Release any fears, worries and concerns you have, knowing that you are being protected and guided by the universe.

## *Number 1515 or 5151*

Universal Number 1515 brings a message of change or changes in your life. This sign guides you in knowing that the changes happening are there for your greater good and to enrich your life moving forward. It is important that you keep your thoughts, words and actions in a positive mindset. Any thoughts of fear or worries can impact the outcome of these changes.

## *Number 1616 or 6161*

The number 6 together with the number 1 brings a message of worry regarding financial matters or material concerns. This is a message from the universe to focus on more important matters, such as family issues, your home life and you as an individual. Keep your thoughts positive and let go of any fears regarding your career, finances and other material matters.

## *Number 1717 or 7171*

Number 1717 is a sign that you have an important life purpose that will inspire and teach others. You are being guided to use your unique talents to better serve humanity through your words and actions. Your positive actions set an inspiring example to others. Ensure that you keep up this good work and continue to be a beacon of light.

### Number 1818 or 8181

Universal Number sequence 1818 is a positive message of abundance. This is a sign that your thoughts and prayers have been heard and will be answered. The universe is letting you know that you will receive an increased flow of abundance in your life, whether this comes in the form of financial, emotional, spiritual or physical abundance.

### Number 1919 or 9191

This number suggests that a phase or situation in your life is coming to a close. The universe is making you aware that the changes happening in your life are for your greater benefit and will positively better your life situation. It is possible that change can come in the way of a career move, financial gain, a relationship and more. Have faith and trust that everything you need will be made available to you on your path by the Universal Energies.

### Number 2323 or 3232

Universal Number sequence 2323 is a message from the universe to keep your thoughts positive about what lies ahead of you on your life path. You are guided to remain centred and balanced in your faith and use positive affirmations to help maintain a positive attitude. Focus on your future successes in your life and visualise all of your wants and desires.

### Bonus Number – Number 123

Number 123 brings you a message to simplify your life and

throw out anything that is unnecessarily using your energy, time or finances. This is a message to clear out the old that is no longer positively serving you and progress forward with clarity of mind and focus.

## *Bonus Number – Number 1234*

Universal Number 1234 brings a similar message to that of 123, but with the addition of the number 4 vibration, the message alters. Number sequence 1234 brings a message of 'steps', stepping forward, action and progression. This is a call to step forward in your life and follow your intuition. Have faith and trust in yourself.

# Emotional Intelligence:
# The Key To Understanding
# Who We Are

*Recognising our own feelings and those of others, motivating ourselves,*
*managing emotions well in ourselves and in our relationships.*
Daniel Goleman on the key to Emotional Intelligence

# Emotional Intelligence: The Importance Of Emotional Intelligence

Intelligence in the human world is often associated with our Intelligence Quotient (IQ), which is our capacity to learn, apply knowledge and solve problems in everyday life, something that many people are familiar with. This is not the only type of intelligence; we also have Emotional Intelligence, which can be known as EQ.

While IQ is still considered as one of the strongest metrics of intelligence, both on a professional and educational level, it is understood that a human being's IQ will only change a small amount from childhood to adulthood. On the other hand, Emotional Intelligence is something that is not automatically in the human psyche and can therefore be learnt at any age.

Becoming a master of Emotional Intelligence takes time, patience and plenty of self-understanding and improvement. EQ is not something someone is able to study, learn and practise overnight to become proficient. EQ is something that needs to be worked on and progressed everyday through critical self-evaluation, a commitment to self-improvement and a commitment to altering your behavioural patterns and psyche.

Emotional Intelligence is an understanding of self, and others, that genuinely sets people apart, especially in a professional environment. Most, if not all, successful leaders have a vast amount of EQ. It is also worth noting that EQ does not necessarily increase with age; those that continue their self-assessment and self-improvement will develop, while those that do not, will not.

## What Is Emotional Intelligence?

Emotional Intelligence has been described in a number of ways. The key to EQ is the ability to recognise, understand and manage emotions in ourselves, and in others. Emotional Intelligence is split into four different sections: Self-Awareness, Self-Management, Social Awareness and Relationship Management.

Emotional Intelligence plays an important role in how we manage behaviour, navigate social complexities and make personal decisions that achieve the required positive results.

In 1995 Daniel Goleman popularised Emotional Intelligence with the release of his book *Emotional Intelligence: Why It Can Matter More Than IQ*. At the time of publication, it was seen as the missing link in a unique finding: people with average IQs outperforming those with the highest IQs 70% of the time.

### *What Is It To Be Emotionally Intelligent?*

A person with high emotional intelligence can and will exhibit these traits:

- The ability to perceive their emotions
- The ability to perceive the emotions of others
- The ability to regulate/manage their emotions
- The ability to regulate/manage the emotions of others
- The ability to understand their gut feeling or intuition
- The ability to understand the emotions of others with a view to building relationships

When we are born, we will naturally inherit Emotional Intelligence; however, by improving our EQ behaviours, the brain will adapt to making these behaviours automatic.

## Where Did It All Begin?

While EQ has been around for an eternity, it has only recently started to be extensively researched and developed. In the 1970s two sets of psychologists, first Howard Gardner (Harvard), who developed the *multiple intelligence* theory, and then with John D. Mayer (New Hampshire) and Peter Salovey (Yale), with the assistance of David R. Caruso, developed Emotional and Social Intelligence or ESI. Their works have been constantly updated, and in the 1990s they first coined the term 'Emotional Intelligence'.

In the 1980s Reuven Bar-On, an Israeli psychologist, developed his theory on emotional intelligence and is acknowledged as one of the leading theorists, researchers and practitioners in this field. The 'Bar-On model of emotional intelligence' is described, in the *Encyclopedia of Applied Psychology*, as one of three leading approaches to this construct.

It was not until a book called *Emotional Intelligence: Why It Can Matter More Than IQ* by Daniel Goleman in 1995 that EQ was popularised and viewed as prominently as IQ. *Emotional Intelligence* was named as one of the 25 *Most Influential Business Management Books* by *TIME Magazine, and the Harvard Business Review* called Emotional Intelligence 'a revolutionary, paradigm-shattering idea'.

In this book, we will look at all three theories of Emotional Intelligence; however, we will focus on the theory of Daniel Goleman. Goleman's theory was the touchpaper that set the topic alight and is usually referred to as the go-to starting point for understanding Emotional Intelligence.

*Recognising our own feelings and those of others, motivating ourselves, managing emotions well in ourselves and in our relationships.*
Daniel Goleman on the key to Emotional Intelligence

# The History Of Emotional Intelligence

**1930**

Edward Thorndike

Components of Social Intelligence

**1940**

David Wechsler

Components of Intelligence

**1950**

Abraham Maslow

Emotional Strength

**1975**

Howard Gardner

Introduces the concept of 'Multiple Intelligence'

**1985**

Reuven Bar-On

Coined the term 'EQ' ('Emotional Quotient') and created the
Bar-On Emotional Quotient Inventory™ (the EQ-i™)

**1985**

Wayne Payne

Introduces the term 'Emotional Intelligence'

**1987**

Keith Beasley

Uses the term 'Emotional Quotient'

**1990**

Peter Salovey and John Mayer

Publish article 'Emotional Intelligence'

**1995**

Daniel Goleman

*Emotional Intelligence: Why It Can Matter More Than IQ*

## Emotional Intelligence And Leadership

Emotional Intelligence is a key driver in leaders and CEOs in professional settings. Emotional Intelligence accounts for 80%-90% of what sets high performers apart from those with similar technical skills and knowledge bases. EQ is constantly used and discussed with regards to leadership and management. It is seen as the key indicator to those who will progress and those that have successfully progressed within their careers and lives to a position of responsibility and much more.

IQ and technical skills are the entry-level requirements for executive positions. EQ is what really separates the high achievers and senior managers from the rest. If you aspire to be in a leadership role, there is an emotional element you must make time to explore and improve. It is, in essence, what helps you successfully coach teams, manage stress, deliver feedback and collaborate with others.

In 1998, Daniel Goleman published an article in the *Harvard Business Review*, 'What Makes a Leader'. He states unequivocally:

*The most effective leaders are all alike in one crucial way: they all have a high degree of what has come to be known as emotional intelligence. It's not that IQ and technical skills are irrelevant. They do matter, but…they are the entry-level requirements for executive positions.*

*My research, along with other recent studies, clearly shows that emotional intelligence is the sine qua non of leadership. Without it, a person can have the best training in the world, an incisive, analytical mind and an endless supply of smart ideas, but he still won't make a great leader.*

## What Does The Science Suggest?

There have been many surveys undertaken and research conducted within the workplace regarding Emotional Intelligence. Research made available by US EQ provider TalentSmart has shown that Emotional Intelligence is to be viewed as the strongest predictor of performance. From the data collated, it seems that more hiring managers are giving greater focus to EQ.

In a survey conducted by US firm CareerBuilder, they found that 71% of employers surveyed said that they valued EQ over IQ. They also found that employees with high emotional intelligence were more likely to stay calm under pressure, resolve conflict effectively and respond to co-workers with empathy. In their concluding finding, those surveyed said that employees with a higher level of EQ were in the top quartile to be promoted every time.

US EQ provider TalentSmart assessed Emotional Intelligence next to 33 other crucial workplace skills, and found that it is the strongest predictor of performance. The data went on to show that a high level of Emotional Intelligence resulted in successful career outcomes 58% of the time across all industries.

*If your emotional abilities aren't in hand, if you don't have self-awareness, if you are not able to manage your distressing emotions, if you can't have empathy and have effective relationships, then no matter how smart you are, you are not going to get very far.*
Daniel Goleman

# The Three Major Theories That Gave Birth To Emotional Intelligence

## John Mayer And Peter Salovey's Ability Model

In the 1970s John Mayer and Peter Salovey developed their four cornerstones of Emotional Intelligence; these were later updated with the development of Emotional Intelligence and the research behind it. The four cornerstones are:

PERCEPTION
FACILITATION
UNDERSTANDING
MANAGEMENT/REGULATION

**Perception** – the ability to perceive emotions in yourself, others and in the environment around you

**Facilitation** – the ability to use emotion/s to interpret the world and facilitate thought

**Understanding** – the ability to understand emotions, emotional language and emotional signals, as well as applying words and knowledge to the emotions

**Management/Regulation** – the ability to manage/control your emotions and those of your peers with a specific goal in mind

## Reuven Bar-On's Competencies Model

Reuven Bar-On, Israeli psychologist, wrote about Emotional Intelligence and his EQ-i assessment method in various publications from 1982. In his original theory, Bar-On believes the five cornerstones of Emotional Intelligence are:

INTERPERSONAL
DECISION-MAKING
SELF-EXPRESSION
SELF-PARTICIPATION
STRESS MANAGEMENT

They are divided into 15 representative subdivisions:

**Interpersonal** – interpersonal relationships, empathy, social responsibility

**Decision-Making** – problem-solving, reality testing, impulse control

**Self-Expression** – emotional expression, assertiveness, independence

**Self-Participation** – self-regard, self-actualisation, emotional self-awareness

**Stress Management** – flexibility, stress tolerance, optimism

## Daniel Goleman's Performance Model

In Daniel Goleman's 1995 book *Emotional Intelligence: Why It Can Matter More Than IQ*, he believes the four cornerstones of Emotional Intelligence are:

SELF-AWARENESS
SELF-MANAGEMENT
EMPATHY AND SOCIAL AWARENESS
RELATIONSHIP MANAGEMENT

**Self-Awareness** – knowing/understanding your internal states, preferences, resources and intuitions

**Self-Management** – managing your internal states, impulses and resources

**Social Awareness and Empathy** – how people handle relationships and the awareness of others' feelings, needs and concerns

**Relationship Management** – the skill or adeptness at inducing desirable responses in others

*What really matters for success, character, happiness and lifelong achievements is a definite set of emotional skills – your EQ – not just purely cognitive abilities that are measured by conventional IQ tests.*
Daniel Goleman

# Daniel Goleman's Emotional Intelligence

Goleman's four cornerstones of Emotional Intelligence are:

Self-Awareness
Self-Management
Empathy And Social Awareness
Relationship Management

## Self-Awareness

Self-Awareness is key to Goleman's theory. It is the ability to accurately recognise your emotions, abilities, limitations, actions and goals, and understand how these affect you and those around you. Self-awareness is at the very core of everything and is the main element of Emotional Intelligence.

Self-awareness is comprised of three competencies:

**Emotional Self-Awareness** – is where you are able to read and understand your emotions, and at the same time recognise their impact on your work performance and relationships

**Accurate Self-Assessment** – is where you are able to give a realistic evaluation of your strengths, weaknesses and limitations

**Self-Confidence** – is where you have a positive opinion of yourself and a strong sense of your self-worth. The focus and entrance point in these areas is the ability to be critically self-reflective

# Self-Management

Self-Management is the ability for you to manage your emotions and impulses in difficult or stressful situations, and maintain a positive outlook despite setbacks. Those who lack self-management tend to react and have a harder time keeping their impulses in check.
Self-management is comprised of six competencies:

**Emotional Self-Control** – is keeping disruptive emotions and impulses under control

**Transparency** – is maintaining standards of trustworthiness, honesty and integrity, managing yourself and responsibilities

**Adaptability** – is the flexibility in adapting to changing situations and overcoming obstacles

**Achievement** – is the guiding drive and determination to meet an internal standard of excellence

**Initiative** – is the readiness to seize opportunities and take action (today)

**Optimism** – is persistence in pursuing goals despite obstacles and setbacks

## Social Awareness And Empathy

While it is important to be aware of yourself, it is also a vital skill to be aware of others and empathetically understanding towards them. Social awareness describes the ability to recognise emotions in others and the atmosphere of a situation, room or company.

Social Awareness is comprised of three competencies:

**Empathy** – is understanding others and taking an active interest in their worries and concerns

**Awareness** – is the ability to read the currents and trends of organisational life, build decision networks and navigate politics

**Service Orientation** – is recognising, understanding and meeting customers' needs

# Relationship Management

Relationship management refers to the ability to influence, coach and mentor others, and resolve conflict effectively. While most people prefer to stay clear of conflict, in a position of leadership being able to embrace those conversations is a wonderful skill. Relationship management is comprised of 7 competencies:

**Visionary Leadership** – is inspiring and guiding groups of people and individuals

**Developing Others** – is the propensity to develop, strengthen and support the abilities of others through feedback and guidance

**Influence** – is the ability to exercise a wide range of persuasive strategies with integrity; sending clear, convincing and well-tuned messages. This also includes listening

**Change Catalyst** – is proficiency in implementing new ideas and guiding people in a new direction

**Conflict Management** – is resolving disagreements and collaboratively developing resolutions

**Building Bonds** – is building and maintaining relationships with others

**Teamwork and Collaboration** – are the promotion of cooperation and building of teams

# Daniel Goleman's Emotional Intelligence In Practice

## *Emotional Intelligence In Life*

Emotional Intelligence is an important aspect of our make-up and how we live our daily lives, whether this is personally or professionally. Within our careers, many businesses and organisations will assess and look to assist in developing their staff by using the lessons within the Emotional Intelligence framework. The principles behind EQ provide a different vantage point when understanding and assessing the behaviour, attitudes, motivation, interpersonal skills, future potential and management styles of people in an organisation.

Emotional Intelligence is now commonplace within human resources departments worldwide. EQ is used for management development, the interview and hiring process, resources planning, customer relations, etc. EQ plays a vital role in almost all areas of our lives.

Research conducted by Tasha Eurich PhD, organisational psychologist and *New York Times* bestselling author, states that 95% of people believe they are self-aware; however, the actual number of self-aware people is in the region of 10%-15%, quite a dramatic difference. In a survey conducted by Eurich across differing industries, she found that of those surveyed, 99% said that they worked with someone who was not self-aware. Of those 99%, 73% were colleagues, 33% were direct line managers, 32% were bosses and 16% were clients.

Eurich's research on self-awareness highlights that working alongside colleagues who are not self-aware can lead to a reduction in the success of the team, or company, by up to 50%. In addition to this, Eurich's research suggests that working with those who lack self-awareness can increase stress and employee turnover, as well as decreasing motivation. The same theory can also be applied to anyone in your life that is not self-aware. They are likely to cause you increased stress, demotivation and a breakdown in relations with that person. Of course, in a workplace you have less of a choice with your colleagues than you would have with your circle of friends. Families can be another matter.

Leaders set the culture and rhythm of their business.

Should they be lacking in emotional intelligence, it is highly likely to have more far-reaching and negative consequences. When you have a leader, boss or partner who lacks in EQ it often results in lower employee engagement, higher staff turnover and a poor, if not toxic, workplace environment.

While it is possible that someone may have strong technical skills, if they are unable to communicate with others effectively and efficiently, those technical skills become less relevant. Spending time to master the skills of Emotional Intelligence will not only advance your career or company, it will also have dramatic positive effects on your daily life with all those you interact with, bringing you more joy, contentment and understanding in your life.

# Four Cornerstones, Five Skills:
# How To Use EQ For Your Own Benefit

As mentioned previously, Daniel Goleman published an article in the *Harvard Business Review*, 'What Makes a Leader'.

In this article he identified five main skills of Emotional Intelligence; these are:

Self-Awareness
Self-Regulation
Empathy
Social Skills
Motivation

**Self-Awareness** – is knowing your own strengths, weaknesses, moods, drives, aspirations, values and their impact on others

**Self-Regulation** – is controlling, managing or redirecting disruptive impulses and moods

**Empathy** – is understanding other people's emotional make-up and considering their feelings, especially when making decisions

**Social Skills** – are building rapport with others to move them in a desired direction, an ability to find common ground

**Motivation** – is relishing achievement and being driven for its own sake

# Self-Awareness

*The ability to recognise and understand your moods, emotions and drives, as well as their effect on others.*

## *Key Factors In Determining Self-Awareness*

- Self-confidence
- Emotional awareness
- Accurate and realistic self-assessment
- Self-deprecating sense of humour
- Thirst for constructive criticism

## *Benefits Of Being Self-Aware*

- Able to manage and use constructive feedback effectively
- Knowing your strengths, weaknesses and abilities
- Knowing who you are on an emotional level
- Understanding your key drivers and desires
- Understanding your core emotional triggers

## *Self-Awareness Is The Key To Emotional Intelligence*

Richard Boyaztis and Michelle Burckle, Emotional Intelligence theorists and creators of one of the most recognised Emotional Intelligence tests, suggest:

- With self-awareness a person has a 49% chance of demonstrating self-management
- Without self-awareness a person has a 4% chance of demonstrating self-management
- With self-awareness a person has a 38% chance of demonstrating social awareness

- Without self-awareness a person has a 17% chance of demonstrating social awareness

In an article in the *Harvard Business Review* focused on self-awareness, Erich Dierdorff and Robert Rubin revealed that teams or units with a collectively high level of self-awareness outperform teams with low self-awareness. In fact, those teams with high self-awareness outperform across decision-making, coordination and conflict management.

- With high self-awareness a team has a 68% probability of being successful in making a quality decision
- With low self-awareness a team has a 32% probability of being successful in making a quality decision
- With high self-awareness a team has a 73% probability of engaging in successful team coordination
- With low self-awareness a team has a 27% probability of engaging in successful team coordination
- With high self-awareness a team has a 65% probability of engaging in successful conflict management
- With low self-awareness a team has a 35% probability of engaging in successful conflict management

## *How To Improve Self-Awareness*

- Spend time getting to know and understand yourself (meditation and contemplation)
- Keep a diary of the situations that have triggered negative emotions in you. At this time, note your thoughts and behaviours during those situations
- Ask for a 360-degree review or ask for feedback from colleagues, friends, employers…
- Observe the response others have to your behaviour

# Self-Regulation

*The ability to control or redirect disruptive impulses and moods, and the propensity to suspend judgement – to think before acting.*

### Key Factors In Determining Self-Regulation

- Self-control
- Conscientiousness
- Trustworthiness
- Adaptability
- Innovation
- Integrity
- Comfort with ambiguity
- Reliability

### Benefits Of Being Self-Regulated

- Ability to keep negative emotions under control
- Assists in helping to earn the respect and trust of others
- Ability to adapt to change with minimal fuss
- Allows you to have a brighter and more positive outlook

### How To Improve Self-Regulation

- Accepting blame and not passing the blame onto others
- Taking responsibility for errors or mistakes made
- Responding to a situation with a level head
- Use your communication in an effective and calm state
- Practising breathing techniques, such as controlled breathing, can be useful
- Remember to pause, breathe, collect yourself and do whatever it takes to manage your emotions

# Motivation

*A passion to work for reasons that go beyond money or status, and a propensity to pursue goals with energy and persistence.*

## Key Factors In Determining Motivation

- Achievement drive
- Commitment
- Initiative
- Optimism
- Passion
- Focus
- Energy

## Benefits Of Being Motivated

- Encourages less procrastination when decision-making
- Ability to feel and be more self-confident
- Having courage in the face of adversity
- Having a passion to succeed
- Ability to be focused on your goals and aspirations
- Motivation is infectious and can motivate others

## How To Improve Your Motivation

- Understand your 'why', know why you started this journey
- Find new targets and goals to achieve
- Keep challenging yourself and do not rest on your laurels
- Keep a positive and optimistic mindset, find the positives in even the most challenging of situations

# Empathy

*The ability to understand the emotional make-up of other people, and the skill in treating people according to their emotional reactions.*

## Key Factors In Determining Empathy

- Service orientation
- Developing others
- Leveraging diversity
- Political awareness
- Expertise in attracting and retaining talent
- Ability to develop and teach others
- Sensitivity to cross-cultural differences
- Strong interpersonal skills

## Benefits Of Being Empathetic

- Assists in understanding other people's emotions
- Assists in the ability to help someone
- Become more compassionate and understanding
- Especially helpful when delivering constructive feedback
- Assists in a positive career working with others
- People will respect you more

## How To Develop Empathy

- Imagine yourself in someone else's position
- Practise listening to people without interrupting them
- Observe those around you and how they are feeling
- Try to understand before forming judgements
- Keep your body language open and regulate your voice to show your sincerity

# Social Skills

*Proficiency in managing relationships and building networks, and an ability to find common ground and build rapport.*

## Key Factors In Determining Social Skills

- Influence
- Communication
- Leadership
- Conflict management
- Building bonds
- Collaboration and cooperation
- Active listening
- Persuasiveness

## Benefits Of Having Social Skills

- Ability to create rapport and build lasting relationships
- Ability to persuade others in a direction of your choosing
- Assists in earning the respect and loyalty of others
- Having an extensive network of contacts
- Expertise in building and leading teams
- Ability to assist others, being more approachable

## How To Improve Social Skills

- Develop your communication skills
- Work on your body language, be more approachable
- Learn how to provide praise and constructive feedback
- Listen to others and practise empathy
- Build relationships with your employees and colleagues
- Look at the situation from all the viewpoints involved

# Qualities Of The Emotionally Intelligent

This can either be used as a checklist for you to improve your own Emotional Intelligence, or something you can use to notice it in others. Are you or the person you are assessing:

- Empathetic
- Self-Aware
- Curious
- Analytically minded
- Passionate
- Optimistic
- Adaptable
- Have belief (faith)
- Have needs and wants
- Have a desire to help others succeed and succeed for yourself

In everyday life, do you or the person you are assessing:

- Think about feelings or emotions
- Take time to pause
- Strive to control your thoughts
- Benefit from criticism
- Show authenticity
- Demonstrate empathy
- Praise others
- Give helpful feedback
- Apologise for mistakes
- Forgive and forget
- Keep your commitments
- Help others
- Say NO often and set boundaries

# What Are Some Of The Benefits
# Of Having A High EQ?

- Ability to be innovative
- Ability to feel and be more self-confident
- Ability to adapt to change with minimal fuss
- Ability to keep negative emotions under control
- Ability to be focused on your goals and aspirations
- Ability to create rapport and build lasting relationships
- Ability to persuade others in a direction of your choosing
- Ability to assist others personally and professionally
- Ability to make positive and lasting change
- Ability to assess situations and make logical decisions
- Ability to use constructive feedback effectively
- Assists in understanding other people's emotions
- Assists in the ability to help someone
- Assists in helping to earn the respect and trust of others
- Assists in a positive career, working with others
- Allows yourself to have a more positive outlook
- Being more compassionate and understanding
- Being more satisfied within your job and career
- Being more approachable to others
- Encourages less procrastination when decision-making
- Especially helpful when delivering constructive feedback
- Expertise in building and leading teams
- Having an extensive network of contacts
- Having courage in the face of adversity
- Having a passion to succeed
- Having improved productivity and efficiency
- Knowing your strengths, weaknesses and abilities
- Knowing who you are on an emotional level
- Understanding your key drivers
- Understanding your core emotional triggers

# What Are Some Of The Implications Of Having A Low EQ?

- Afraid or worried about change
- Blame others for negative emotions and feelings
- Can be easily irritated
- Can be easily distracted
- Can be chronically distressed
- Can be judgemental
- Can be easily offended
- Can be easily stressed
- Can be burnt out from work
- Can feel under appreciated
- Can lack self-respect
- Can lack self-confidence
- Can lack motivation and drive
- Difficulty coping with sadness and emotional pain
- Do not understand their own emotions
- Does not handle constructive criticism well
- Have a lack of empathy
- Have trouble being assertive or taking charge
- Have a limited emotional vocabulary
- Have little emotion in everyday life
- Have difficulty maintaining relationships
- Have a short fuse and quick emotional reactions
- Hold on to grudges
- Hold on to past errors and mistakes
- Find it difficult to maintain any relationships
- Find it hard to say no to others' requests
- Make assumptions quickly
- Often feel misunderstood
- Unable to control emotions
- Unaware of other people's feelings

# Advanced Body Talk – The Unspoken Language

*If language was given to men to conceal their thoughts, then gesture's purpose was to disclose them.*
John Napier

# Breaking Down The Myths
# Of Body Language

Body language is a key element in how we communicate with each other, and is an important factor in Emotional Intelligence. According to Professor Albert Mehrabian, in his book *Silent Messages* (1972), communication is broken down in to three parts: visual; vocal and tonal; and word-only. Professor Mehrabian found that 93% of all communication is non-verbal, with 55% being visual, 38% vocal and tonal, while word-only makes up 7% of how we communicate.

In this chapter, we are connecting our social awareness and self-awareness of Emotional Intelligence to body language. Using the experience and understanding of former FBI special agent Joe Navarro, from his book *The Dictionary of Body Language,* we are focusing on the major signals of body language on the face (mouth, nose, throat, eyes, hair, forehead) and arms (hands and fingers) as these are the areas of the body we see constantly and which give us a lot of visual information.

With body language, it is vitally important to understand and be aware that a person's 'body language', and the change of that language, only represents that very moment, and a reaction to something happening at that time. This could be a question asked, an action by someone (romantic/aggressive), seeing a partner or lover, being handed an invoice, being handed a bonus cheque, being dumped...etc.

Body language, and the reading of it, is all about timing and noticing the changes and subtleties that are being made in front of you. Remember that body language does not equal 100% factual communication; however, using your skills and experience you can bridge the gap for a better understanding.

Former FBI agent Joe Navarro stresses that there are many misconceptions regarding body language that are completely untrue and hold no scientific or empirical proof. For example, touching of the nose, mouth or clearing your throat is often perceived as a guide that someone is lying. This is untrue and holds no ground. The same applies to when a person's eyes are looking in a certain direction; it is not a sign of a mistruth. It purely means that a person is processing the information and it has no bearing on whether they are telling the truth or not. Humans, by nature, are poor judges at spotting deception.

When you look at non-verbal communication, it is NOT about making a judgement, it is about what that person is transmitting at that very moment. We are all transmitting a message and signals at all times. These come from a number of different sources, including the clothes we choose to wear, how we groom and present ourselves, and also how we carry ourselves. How we stand, where we place our hands and arms, and where we are gazing, all have a story to tell.

Recognising and understanding non-verbal communication in others is a key aspect of Emotional Intelligence and is an important skill to improve in ourselves.

## The Hair And Forehead

The hair, forehead, eyebrows, eyes, nose, lips, ears and chin all communicate in their own way – from general health to emotional distress.

### *Hair*

Our hair conveys so much when it comes to non-verbal communication. All people look for healthy hair, it is one of the first things they notice. If someone has dirty, messy and unhealthy hair, it may suggest that person is suffering from poor health, or even poor mental health. The way in which someone styles and looks after their hair says a lot about them and can give an idea to the career they have.

### *Playing With Hair*

Playing with hair is usually used as a comforting behaviour, also described as a pacifying behaviour. It is typically used by those with longer hair and can either indicate a person being in a good mood or being stressed.

### *Running Fingers Through Hair – Men*

When a man runs his fingers through his hair it is highlighting that he is stressed or worried about a situation. It can denote that a person has doubt or concern.

### *Ventilating Hair – Women*

When upset, worried, stressed or flustered, women tend to lift up their hair at the back of their neck quickly. When this is repeated it is likely that they are overly stressed, unless involved in physical activity.

## Hair Pulling

When someone is repetitively and intentionally pulling out their hair, this is medically referred to as trichotillomania. Hair pulling is a sure sign of stress and is something that occurs in both men and women. Men tend to pluck their eyebrows, while women range from pulling their head hair to plucking their eyebrows, eyelids, arm hair and leg hair.

## Head Nodding

When in a conversation with someone nodding, this is a signal that the other person is listening and receptive to the message. Nodding also is a sign of agreement to what is being communicated.

## Head Scratching

Head scratching is often associated with having doubts or being stressed or frustrated; however, when someone is frantically scratching their head it is usually a sign of panic and being highly stressed.

## Head Scratching With Belly Rub

Head scratching with the simultaneous rubbing of the belly highlights concern, doubt and worry. It is also a sign of insecurity, self-doubt and uncertainty.

## Head Stroking

Stroking our heads is something we do to keep our hair looking presentable. When we are stressed, we can stroke our hair with the palm of the hand as a soothing mechanism. The same can also apply when we are unsure of an answer to a question or unsure about a decision.

## Forehead Furrowing

From the moment of birth we look to the forehead for information, it reveals to others how we are feeling. If someone is furrowing their forehead there is a good chance that there is a problem or that the person is insecure.

## Botoxed Forehead

Botox is a cosmetic procedure that is commonplace with both men and women. When someone has Botox in their forehead it can create a problem for their non-verbal communication, as their forehead has limited movement and cannot offer information into how that person is feeling. This situation can affect personal, professional and family relationships.

## Forehead Stress Lines

The stress lines on a person's forehead that are marked by deep grooves often signal someone who has had struggles or stresses in their life. It can also be a sign of someone who has spent time in the outdoors, or in harsh weather conditions.

## Forehead Sweating

While everyone has their own personal levels of sweating, it is possible that when a person is highly stressed or emotional, they can spontaneously sweat from their forehead. It is important to understand someone's sweat levels before coming to an adjudged conclusion.

## *Forehead Massaging*

When someone massages their forehead it is usually a sign that they are trying to process some information or are worried or anxious. Massaging the forehead is a pacifying and soothing behaviour when stressed or apprehensive.

## The Eyes

Our eyes are vital in so many aspects of our make-up and being. Eyes give away so much about us and how we feel, whether this is showing love, compassion, fear or worry. We naturally use our eyes to attract and avert others. When we want to attract someone, we look into their eyes aiming to connect with them. Whereas when we want to avoid someone, we do all we can to ensure we do not make eye contact. Our eyes are often perceived to be the windows to our soul.

### *Pupil Dilation*

Our eyes give away so much about us. When we like someone or something our pupils dilate. This is a real telltale sign if you are attracted or fancy someone. This is an instinctive action and we have no control over it.

### *Pupil Constriction*

Correspondingly to when our pupils dilate, pupil constriction is an automatic response and happens when we have negative emotions or see something we do not like or enjoy. This happens to ensure that our eyes are focused in times of concern and danger.

### *Relaxed Eyes*

If someone has relaxed eyes it is usually a sign that they themselves are relaxed, comfortable and self-confident. When we are relaxed and comfortable all the muscles in the eyes, cheeks and forehead relax. At a time of stress, the muscles surrounding the eyes offer an almost immediate signal into a person's mental state.

## Frequent Blinking

When someone blinks rapidly it is usually a sign of increased tension, stress or becoming nervous.

We all blink more frequently when heavily questioned; it is therefore not a sign of someone lying.

## Eye Contact

Eye contact is something that changes from culture to culture and is not the same worldwide. In some cultures, it is acceptable to look at someone in the eye for a few seconds, whereas others do not allow this. In the Western world, eye contact is often a sign of confidence, respect and defiance, depending on the situation.

## Eye Avoidance

Avoiding eye contact can mean different things in different circumstances. When we avoid eye contact in a social setting it can mean that a person is shy, embarrassed, has shame or is deliberately avoiding someone. Avoiding eye contact is not a sure sign of deception.

## Gaze Superiority

Global studies have found that people with a high social status engage in more direct eye contact when both speaking and listening. Those with a lower social status are more likely to make eye contact when they are listening, while making less eye contact when they are speaking. This can also be an indication of a lack of self-confidence.

## Closed Eyes

In professional or non-personal situations, the closing or covering of the eyes for a long period of time is associated with worry, concern or disapproval. While in an intimate setting, a person that closes their eyes for a sustained period of time is saying that they trust the other person and want to block out all other possible distractions, so they can focus on who they are spending time with.

## Eyelids Fluttering

Should you observe someone that has a sudden bout of eyelid fluttering it is likely that person is struggling to deal with a situation, or a problem has arisen. Eyelid fluttering can also happen when someone struggles to find an appropriate word when speaking or in conversation.

## Eye Rolling

This is something that most people will be aware of. When a person rolls their eyes, they are communicating disrespect, disapproval and often frustration.

## Looking Sideways

Looking sideways is often connected with a person who is having doubts about a situation and is reluctant to commit to a decision. Looking sideways can portray disbelief and concern.

## Looking Up (Ceiling/Sky)

When someone looks up to the sky or heavens, it is usually associated with an inner cry for help. It can also be connected with disbelief and exasperation.

## *Long Stare*

A long stare, while in a conversation, usually signifies that someone is in deep thought or taking time to process some information. A person in a long stare alone is indicating that they are in deep contemplation and lost in their thoughts.

## The Ears And Nose

The ears and nose both play an important role in our human make-up, especially as they are two of the five senses (hearing and smell). That aside, the ears and nose can communicate many non-verbal signals that can be vital in understanding the subtle messages of others.

### Earlobe Pulling Or Massaging

Earlobe massaging, playing with or pulling are used as soothing pacifiers when a person is stressed or in deep thought. Light pulling or rubbing of the ears is relaxing.

### Ear Blushing

There is a myth that our ears turn bright red, or blush, when someone is thinking or talking about us. The real reason for this to happen is due to a hormonal change in our body. This can be caused by being angry, embarrassed, fearful or anxious.

### Ear Leaning

During a conversation, if someone turns their ear towards the speaker and leans forward, they are showing that they are listening with intent and hanging on every word that person is saying. In a noisy setting, it can mean that a person is struggling to hear or that they are hard of hearing and want something repeated.

### Scarred Or Damaged Ears

There are a number of potential reasons for someone to have damaged ears, including chemicals, trauma or overexposure to extreme weather elements. It is known that rugby players, mixed martial artists, wrestlers and others involved in full-contact sports are susceptible to damaged ears, often described as cauliflower ear/s.

## Covering Nose With Both Hands

When someone covers their nose and mouth simultaneously in a sudden or instant reaction, this usually depicts shock, fear, surprise, disbelief or disturbance. This is something that can happen when we see something that is shocking to us, such as a bad accident, a crime, an act of violence or horror, etc.

## Nose Wrinkling Upwards

The nose wrinkle is usually an indication of dislike, repulsion or disgust. When a person sees, hears or smells something they do not like or are repulsed by, their nasal muscles involuntarily contract.

## Nose Twitching

When a person is looking directly at someone, nose twitching is similar to the nose wrinkle above and can indicate dislike or disgust. The nose twitch is something that is done more rapidly than a wrinkle; it can be as quick as a blink of an eye. In many Caribbean countries, a nose twitch, without squinting eyes, can mean, 'How can I help you?' or 'What's going on?'

## Nostril Flaring

Nostril flaring is something that takes places in preparation for a physical activity or running away from the situation. It is a good indicator that the person flaring their nostrils needs some time to calm down.

## *Long Index Finger To Nose*

A long index finger to the nose or close to the nose for an elongated time period is often associated with someone who is deep in thought, has worries or is concerned about a situation or event.

## *Nose Brushing*

The brushing or lightly rubbing of the nose highlights that a person is either under stress or psychological discomfort. As with the index finger to the nose, brushing the nose can also signal that someone is concerned with something questionable and is in thought.

## *Holding Nose High*

Holding the nose high in an intentional manner is a strong indication of self-confidence, ego, superiority and potentially contempt. Depending on the situation it can also be an aggressive and dismissive action.

## *Nose Tapping*

The tapping of the nose can have two distinctive and different meanings. When someone taps their nose it can indicate that they do not trust the person speaking or that they are closely watching their actions. Conversely, tapping the nose can also communicate that a person thinks the other person is intelligent and that they acknowledge them.

## *Sneaking Nose Touch*

Using the index finger, sneaking a touch of the nose with the lightest of pacifying touches indicates masked/hidden tension.

## *Rapid Nose Inhaling*

Rapid nose inhalation usually takes place before someone is about to give unpleasant or negative news. In many cases, the breathing through the nose is so fast that it is audible before they speak. It can also take place before a lie.

## The Mouth And Lips

The mouth and lips are secondary to the eyes in communicating non-verbal signals. The mouth can register and express an array of emotions, from sadness to ecstasy and everything in between. The mouth and lips can give away much of how we are feeling and what we are thinking.

### Chewing Gum

Chewing gum is something that many people do to ease their nerves, freshen their breath or to assist healthy dental hygiene. When someone chews vigorously it can signal worry or that they are anxious. There have been many professional sports coaches that chewed gum regularly on the sidelines to calm their nerves.

### Dry Mouth

Often described as 'cotton-mouth' or the medical term 'Xerostomia'. Having a dry mouth is brought on by fear, worry and anxiety. Should a person have a dry mouth, it is not an indication that they are lying.

### Yawning

Yawning helps to relieve stress by stimulating the nerves in the jaw and is a great soother and pacifier. Scientifically, yawning cools the blood circulation in the palate of the mouth and the blood to the brain. Therefore, when someone yawns it can be an indication that they are too hot.

### Smoking Or Vaping

Those who smoke or vape often increase the amount they smoke when stressed or under pressure. In many instances when severely stressed, the smoker is completely unaware of the amount they are smoking. This in turn can lead to a number of physical illnesses. When you notice someone smoking continuously it is likely that they are overly stressed and highly pressured.

## Overeating

In a similar vein to a smoker, when someone is under a great deal of stress or pressure, they will overeat to help calm their nerves. At times, it is possible for a person to overeat to the point of being sick.

## Tongue In Cheek

Someone who has pushed their tongue against their cheek and holds it in place is likely to be hiding something or trying to get away with something they have done. It can also mean that a person is in a highly stressful situation.

## Voice Pitch

Our vocal cords tense when we are stressed, nervous or when we feel insecure. This means that when someone is either nervous, stressed or insecure, their voice can raise in tone and crack when speaking.

## Speed Of Talking

The speed at which we speak is a vitally important non-verbal indicator. The tone, accent, speed and pronunciation of someone speaking gives away much information about that person, including where they originate from, their educational level, their personality and more. When there is a change in the usual speed of how someone speaks, it usually indicates stress or a reluctance to answer a specific question.

## Incessant Talking

People who often talk continuously or incessantly are usually nervous and can be unsure of the content they are saying. It can also highlight a lack of Emotional Intelligence, self-awareness and social awareness. When someone is self-confident and speaks without allowing others to participate, it is usually a signal that they believe they are superior to you.

## Coughing Or Clearing Of The Throat

When someone clears their throat or coughs, it is often to answer a question they find tricky or challenging. It is possible that a person may clear their throat when lying or using deception, although this is not a reliable indicator.

## Lip Biting

Should you notice a person biting their lip, it can signify that they are stressed or are worried about something. It can also highlight that someone wants to say something and are holding themselves back for some reason. Biting our lips is a soothing and pacifying action as it stimulates the nerves in our mouth, just as sucking our thumb would.

## Lip Licking (All Around)

Licking our lips has a similar pacifying effect to biting them. We do this when we are anxious, worried, feel sad or upset. Conversely, it is possible that a person is licking their lips because they are dry. This is usually a very good indicator that someone is stressed.

## Upper-Lip Tongue Licking

When you notice a person licking only their upper lip, this is often associated with someone experiencing positive emotions. It is also possible to be used as a stress reliever.

# The Neck

The neck is a critical area of the body as it has a direct influence over the blood supply to the brain, food and water to the stomach, electrical signals from the brain to the rest of the body and the air flow to our lungs. Needless to say, the neck plays a vital role in our survival; however, it is also one of the weakest and most vulnerable areas of our body.

## Neck Touching

Neck touching is a clear guide to how someone is feeling. It highlights that someone is insecure, apprehensive, concerned or anxious. A touch of the neck, no matter how light, is one of the most accurate signs that something is worrying us. This is not the case if someone has an itch to scratch.

## Touching A Tie-Knot/Necklace

Touching either the knot of a tie, or a necklace performs a protective action by defending a vulnerable area (throat) and assists in relieving anxiety and stress through repetitive movement.

## Playing With Shirt Collar

Touching and playing with the collar of a shirt acts as a pacifying and stress-relieving behaviour. By playing with the shirt collar, we are able to ventilate the body and cover/protect the neck area. The repetitive nature of playing with the shirt collar can also act as a pacifying behaviour.

## Neck Massaging

Neck massaging is another clear signal of distress or concern. A person would massage their neck to relieve stress or pain, and to ease tension. A neck massage performed by oneself usually ONLY happens when there is something of concern.

## Skin Pull

Underneath the chin there is an area of flesh and skin that often serves as a pacifier to relax and calm some men. It is a rare occurrence to see this action in women. In times of extreme stress, the pulling of the skin in the neck area can become vigorous, leaving marks, soreness and redness.

## Neck Stretching

The moving of the head and neck in a circular motion is a pacifying action that helps to relieve stress and tension. When being asked a question that a person would prefer not to answer, this action can often be witnessed.

## Neck Exposure

A person will tilt their head to the side, exposing the side of the neck, to indicate that they are listening to someone with interest and giving them their undivided attention. It can also be a sign of showing empathy for someone, and is an excellent way to disarm aggressive behaviour when dealing with confrontation.

## Neck Stiffening

When someone has a stiffened neck during a conversation, especially when initially relaxed, it indicates they either have an important matter to discuss or that they have an issue with what they have heard. A stiffened neck is a sign of being alert and vigilant.

## The Arms

Our arms communicate a lot about how we feel, they are among the most expressive parts of our body. As well as communication, our arms play an important role in our protection, balance and holding what we need in our daily lives. Our arms say a lot about us and how we express ourselves.

### Gesturing While Speaking

Gesturing when speaking is an essential part of non-verbal communication. When we gesture, we do so to emphasise what we are saying, or to try to make ourselves look more believable or likeable. It is also a great way to maintain the attention of others when speaking. Connecting how we gesture to what we are saying is a powerful communicative tool as it enhances our message ten-fold.

### Animated Gestures

When we are animated it is usually a sign that we are expressing our emotions. Animated gestures when speaking are vital to communication, especially when emphasising a point with exaggerated gestures. Being animated is an expressive quality that can tremendously increase a person's success rate in commanding a crowd or audience.

### Arms Held Behind Back

Having our arms behind our back gives a message to others that we want space and not to be overcrowded. This is also often associated with being aloof; it is therefore not recommended to stand this way when meeting with someone for the first time.

## Arm Crossing

Crossing our arms is often perceived to be a blocking or defensive mechanism from the person we are interacting with; this may be correct, depending on the situation. The following highlights that when a person is crossing their arms we need to understand and evaluate the current situation to make an informed assessment.

## Arm Crossing – Self Hugging

When we cross our arms, we often do so to comfort ourselves and are then effectively giving ourselves a hug, a self-hug. We do this when we want to soothe ourselves and it is something we do more in public than in private. For example, if you are in a movie theatre, on an airplane or standing in-line to visit the lavatory. There are many reasons why we cross our arms; do not jump straight to thinking someone is being defensive and protective.

## Arm Crossing – Protection

Someone crossing their arms in protection usually indicates that they are feeling unwell, insecure or vulnerable. It is also possible that when someone is threatened they will close or tighten up, like a clam, for self-protection.

## Arm Crossing – Self-Restraint

A self-restraining hug is very different to a self-hug. Whereas a self-hug is calming, soothing and loving, a self-restraining hug is far more forceful and aggressive. This is a sign of great discomfort and distress. A person is likely to demonstrate facial anguish and strain along with this action.

## *Arm Crossing – Dislike*

Arm crossing when we dislike someone is similar to when we protect ourselves. This protection comes from the dislike of another person and we cross our arms in an attempt to distance and shield ourselves from that person. This action will happen in the moment we see this person, which is why it accurately communicates our dislike for that individual.

## *Arm Crossing – Massaging*

Crossing our arms can be a comfortable position to sit in; however, when someone is crossing their arms and rubbing or massaging their opposite arm or shoulder, this denotes stress, concern, worry or anxiety. This usually occurs when a person is either sitting in a chair or resting their elbows on a surface such as a table.

## *Arm Crossing – Holding Wrist*

Holding our wrist when crossing our arms is an immediate sign of discontent, worry or being in a weak position. This can take place when a person has been given some detrimental information, as well as when being accused of something.

## *Excessive Sweating*

Excessive sweating can happen without an emotional reaction in the body; however, when someone sweats excessively it can highlight that they are under pressure, under stress or hiding something. It is important to understand someone's sweat levels before coming to an adjudged conclusion.

## *Hair Standing On End (Piloerection)*

According to Gavin de Becker in his book *The Gift of Fear*, when we are in a situation or are meeting someone and the hairs on the back of our neck stand up, we must take note as this is a subconscious message that all is not well. Be aware!

## The Hands And Fingers

We use our hands and fingers for almost all of our daily activities; we also communicate with our hands and fingers, especially through signs. Our hands and fingers alone can speak the words of the deaf – that is an amazing form of communication in itself.

### Condition Of Hands

How we groom ourselves is a great indication of how we care for ourselves and our mental wellbeing. Our hands can give away a lot of information depending on the condition of the skin, our nails (long/short, clean/dirty), any scarring or cuts, as well as any physical damage.

### Hand Grooming

If a person has well-groomed hands, it is a sign that they look after their wellbeing and are a mentally and physically healthy person. When we present clean hands, fingers and nails, it highlights to others that we care about ourselves. Those people with chewed or damaged nails, cuts and dirty hands portray that they have a lack of self-care.

### Nail Biting

People who bite their nails are often anxious, worried, insecure or lacking in confidence. When we bite our nails, it is to help relieve tension and worry. In times of great stress, it is possible that we may bite our nails even if we have never done so previously.

## Frequency Of Touching Others

How often we touch others when we are with them is a great way of communicating our emotions without saying a word. While it is possible to show distain or dislike through touch, it is usually the softer gentler touches that express our love or admiration for others. For example, when we are with a partner we will often rub or stroke their back as we pass them. This lightness of touch is enough to send a message that you care and you are close by.

## Touching Connection

When we touch someone a chemical in our body is released, this chemical is called oxytocin. This is a powerful hormone that serves to socially bind us. This is why you will see people of influence shaking hands, gripping an arm, hugging, holding or kissing babies.

## Pushing Away From The Table

This would usually apply to a meeting or conversation sitting around a table or in a boardroom. Should you find yourself in front of someone who suddenly pushes themselves away from the table with a stiff-arm, this is a highly accurate indication that the person feels threatened or vehemently disagrees with what has been said.

## Playing With Objects

Fidgeting or playing with objects such as a pen, smartphone, stress ball, paperclip...etc. serves as a way to soothe and calm ourselves. This is something we often do when we are in a waiting room, waiting in line or waiting for a meeting to begin, just about anywhere we are waiting for something to start and are killing time.

## Hand Steepling

Performing a hand-steeple when speaking is a clear indication that a person has a high level of self-confidence. When someone performs a hand-steeple they are demonstrating that they have complete and utter belief in what they are saying/presenting. That said, this does not indicate the accuracy of what a person is saying, only the fact that they have complete confidence in themselves. A hand-steeple is created when a person places the fingertips of both hands together and spreads them like a church steeple.

## Interlaced Steepling

The steeple can take different forms; however, the message remains consistent. When you see someone performing a hand-steeple with interlaced fingers, they are demonstrating confidence and self-belief.

## Palms-Up Display

Palms up or hands up is a certain signal of a person saying that they will comply, a sign of submission or that they want to be trusted and believed. When we are speaking and display the palms of our hands, it is a sign to say that you are open, have nothing to hide and that your hands are clean (you can trust me).

## Palms-Down Display

Palms-down is usually displayed on a table or surface, although it can be done in mid-air. The action of a person bringing the palms of their hands down firmly (on a table) is usually coupled with a statement professing or pleading their innocence. The more firmly a person brings their hands to a surface, the more likely it is that they are telling the truth.

## Hand Restriction

It has been researched by applied social psychologist Aldert Vrij that humans tend to move around less when they lie. Therefore, when a person's hand or arm movement becomes restricted when speaking, it is likely that they are lying.

## Finger Holding

Holding our fingers is a pacifying technique we use when we are feeling insecure; it makes us feel more comfortable and at ease. When we hold our fingers, it is not something that we hide and is often associated with when we meet people for the first time.

## Interlaced Fingers-Thumbs Up

We interlace our fingers and thumbs, usually placed on a table or our laps, to emphasise what we are saying. When we raise our thumbs, and possibly move our hands forward, it demonstrates self-confidence and commitment to what we are saying.

## Self-Touching When Answering

Those who touch, rub or stroke themselves when answering a question are using a pacifying technique as they feel uncomfortable, insecure or lack confidence in what they are saying. Those who use their hands to highlight what they are communicating are usually far more confident.

## Surrogate Touching

Surrogate touching is when we touch ourselves or another object rather than touching the person we are with. This can take place when we are not comfortable enough with the other person or confident about their reaction to us being intimate or physically touching them. For example, stroking or rubbing our arm or the stem of a glass. This is also a form of flirtatious behaviour.

## Finger Pointing

Finger pointing is often associated with either being in trouble or aggressive behaviour. No one enjoys being pointed at, even when being directed. It is best to use the full hand with fingers together for a less aggressive approach.

## Rubbing Hands On Palms

When we rub our hand and fingers over the palm of our other hand, we usually do this as a calming or soothing action. If this action is increased and done with force, it can be a sign of anguish, stress and worry.

## Tepee Finger Rub

When we interlace our fingers and move them back and forth, we do so to pacify ourselves and to keep us calm. When we recognise others interlacing their fingers and rubbing them together, it is a strong indicator that they are scared, stressed, worried and anxious. This action is usually reserved for situations that are especially negative and stressful.

## *Preening*

Preening, or smartening ourselves up, is something most of us do ahead of meeting with someone that we either want to impress or present the best version of ourselves to. Preening can take many forms; however, the preening of the hair is very common, especially when romantically involved with someone.

## *Preening (Dismissive)*

Preening can be a negative and dismissive action, especially when cleaning or picking one's nails while speaking with someone or at a dinner table. Any person who is more interested in preening themselves than listening, or speaking, to whom they are with is being disrespectful, and is showing contempt for the other person.

# Blink: Seeing Is Really Believing

*In the blink of an eye, a single expert can usually tell you more than a mountain of survey data.*
Malcolm Gladwell

# Blink, You Know More Than You Know

We have already touched upon our gut instincts and our intuition in various chapters of the book thus far. However, is it possible that our gut instincts can be a better guide to us in our daily lives than hours of procrastination, analysis and research? According to Malcolm Gladwell (author and journalist), this is possible for an experienced person or expert using 'thin-slicing' and Rapid Cognition. Thinking fast!

The idea behind Gladwell's *Blink: The Power of Thinking Without Thinking* is that those individuals who are experienced in a certain field will have immediate and reactive gut and physical reactions to a situation, person or item. It is my belief that anyone can have these gut reactions, although it is important to understand what these reactions mean to fully comprehend the messages of the subconscious.

The ability to understand the physical reactions we can experience in a blink of an eye is an essential tool for our Emotional Intelligence, especially social awareness, empathy and self-awareness. Thin-slicing, as Gladwell puts it, is about those first seconds of reading a person's face, body language, the room or a situation – it is subconsciously being aware of everything that is around us and subconsciously delivering any messages to ourselves physically. This is especially heightened when there is a problem or if there is danger around us.

In a similar vein to the rule of 10,000 hours, which was popularised by Gladwell in his bestselling book *Outliers: The Story of Success*, whereby anyone can become an expert of anything with 10,000 hours of practice, Gladwell believes that when someone is an expert with extensive experience, 'There can be as much value in the blink of an eye as in months of rational analysis,' and, 'When we become expert in something, our tastes grow more esoteric and complex.'

## A Snapshot Is Sometimes All You Need

*Anyone who has ever scanned the bookshelves of a new girlfriend or boyfriend – or peeked inside his or her medicine cabinet – understands this implicitly; you can learn as much, or more, from one glance at a private space as you can from hours of exposure to a public face.*

Peeking behind the curtain of someone's personal space often gives strong indications of the type of person they might be. You could tell whether they were messy, what interests they have, whether they look after themselves, have any health concerns etc. Therefore, it is possible to conceive that a snapshot, or 'thin-slicing', is sometimes all we need to make an informed decision regarding a person, situation or event.

## When You Know, You Know!

*Our world requires that decisions be sourced and footnoted, and if we say how we feel, we must also be prepared to elaborate on why we feel that way...We need to respect the fact that it is possible to know without knowing why we know and accept that, sometimes, we're better off that way.*

Throughout our lives it is highly likely that every person will, at some stage, have a strong gut feeling or gut instinct. The gut instinct uses all of our experiences that we have had in our lifetime and sends us a physical signal to inform us that there is something to be aware of. This instinct is rarely, if ever, inaccurate. It is the interpretation that can lead to error.

When you have a feeling that you 'know' something, the chances are that you probably do. The more time you spend learning and understanding about your physical gut reactions, the more they will assist you throughout your life.

## All The Answers Are Locked Away

*Our unconscious reactions come out of a locked room, and we can't look inside that room. Guided by experience a person can become expert.*

Unlike our brains, we are unable to tap into or think with our gut instinct and subconscious mind, we can only be guided by these reactions at any one specific moment. When the feeling or reaction fades, the reason for the reactions also fades with it. Our subconscious is a locked room that cannot be accessed, it is only in a moment of revelation that we can have access to our subconscious or our intuition.

## In The Blink Of An Eye

*In the blink of an eye, a single expert can usually tell you more than a mountain of survey data.*

With extended experience or expertise in a given field, it is possible for a person to give instantaneous knowledge and understanding to a subject or question, in what would otherwise take many hours, weeks or months to research.

A person who has studied, worked regularly and experienced many reoccurring patterns, shapes, numbers...in a specific field or fields will have a heightened gut reaction to anything in their specialised world that seems to be amiss or incorrect. This speaks volumes for having experienced people in the workplace.

## Expertise Is Seeing What Is Not There To See

*Often a sign of expertise is noticing what doesn't happen.*

Seeing what is not seen by others is a key skill in many professions, and used in everyday life. It is looking over a set of financial accounts for the first time, walking into an office, a manufacturing line, a building site, a restaurant...etc. and seeing what isn't there, and usually what is needed.

## Blink With Extensive Deucation and Experience

*Being able to act intelligently and instinctively in the moment is possible only after a long and rigorous course of education and experience.*

Gladwell is adamant that using our gut instincts can be as useful and accurate as many hours' worth of analysis, as long as you have had an extensive education, a long career and that you have detailed knowledge of your subject matter.

Gladwell emphasises that it is not possible to have an accurate gut instinct unless you have great experience. This same theory can be related to the experiences of everyday life and the reactions we experience. Thinking before reacting is still key. Acknowledge your instincts, think, then react.

## Successful Action Is About Balance

*Truly successful decision-making relies on a balance between deliberate and instinctive thinking.*

Utilising the subconscious mind along with the conscious mind is a sure-fire way to ensure that we are making the best and most accurate decisions for ourselves in any circumstance. As our gut reactions are instantaneous and are in need of some decoding, it is therefore important to take a moment to view the subconscious reaction objectively and act in an appropriate manner using deliberate thinking.

This is an important factor of Emotional Intelligence, specifically self-awareness.

## The Answers Are Gone In The Blink Of An Eye

*Insight is not a lightbulb that goes off inside our heads. It is a flickering candle that can easily be snuffed out.*

Our instincts and reactions are not things that we can hold onto for an extended period of time, they can often be fleeting. This is a further reason why it is important to use deliberate thinking alongside instinctive thinking, as it will ensure that the physical reactions and messages are understood correctly, and can be held by the conscious mind for an action to take place.

## When To 'Blink' And When To Think

*When should we trust our instincts, and when should we consciously think things through?*

Within our lives, our instincts play a vital role in keeping us safe and well, that is their key function. Our intuition and instincts should be used at all times; however, it is important that we should question our own instincts to ensure that we are making the correct decisions in the moment before we act or react.

With a greater understanding of self, and self-awareness, it is to be expected that we will become more confident in trusting our instincts and utilising them in our everyday lives.

## Think When Thinking And Think When Feeling

*I think that the task of figuring out how to combine the best of conscious deliberation and instinctive judgement is one of the great challenges of our time.*

Being able to combine conscious deliberation and instinctive judgement is something that can be learnt and exercised over time. In a similar manner to that of Emotional Intelligence, spending time to understand ourselves, our emotions and our reactions will ensure that we not only improve our Emotional Intelligence, we also improve our decision-making skills in our professional careers and daily lives.

## Learning By Example And Direct Experience

*We learn by example and by direct experience because there are real limits to the adequacy of verbal instruction.*

What Gladwell is highlighting with this quote is something that we have touched upon already; that verbal communication only accounts for 45% of how we communicate, with 38% being vocal and tonal, and word-only making up 7%. Thus, making it more difficult to learn practical skills from a classroom or theoretical method.

Learning by having hands-on experience is crucial in learning any skill, whether this is playing an instrument, learning to use machinery or even learning to drive a car. Anyone can read all the textbooks available to us on a specific subject; however, that does not mean they will be successful when putting it into practice. With direct experience and learning by example, we retain far more information and subconsciously develop the skill, rather than the theory.

### Sometimes, Just Sometimes...

*We have, as human beings, a storytelling problem. We're a bit too quick to come up with explanations for things we don't really have an explanation for.*

Sometimes, just sometimes, we know without knowing. We feel the right decisions to make and we understand what path to take. We are connected to our subconscious that just knows. It knows without our conscious mind knowing or understanding why. Sometimes, just sometimes, we don't need to explain the answer or reasoning for a decision. Sometimes, just sometimes, we can 'feel' the answers without needing to know more. Trust in yourself, and your intuition.

# The Five Cornerstones Of
# A Controlled, Happy
# And Contented Life

*If you are impeccable with your word, if you don't take anything personally, if you don't make assumptions, if you always do your best, then you are going to have a beautiful life.*
Don Miguel Ruiz

# Understanding Toltec Wisdom

The understanding of self and raising our self-awareness is a key skill of Emotional Intelligence. Utilising the tools of *The Four Agreements* by Don Miguel Ruiz and *The Fifth Agreements* by Don Miguel Ruiz and Jose Ruiz, I have outlined some key messages and skills that can be used in daily life, and how they can literally give us complete control over our lives.

Don Ruiz's beliefs are based on an ancient Toltec wisdom that has been passed down from generation to generation. Don Ruiz believes that we are all restricted by self-limiting beliefs that hold us back and cause pain, hurt and suffering. By releasing these self-limiting beliefs, we are able to transform our lives and experience true happiness, freedom and love.

Don Miguel says that:

*It was not your choice to speak English. You didn't choose your religion or your moral values – they were already there before you were born. We never had the opportunity to choose what to believe or what not to believe. We never chose even the smallest of these agreements. We didn't even choose our own name.*

His belief is that from birth we are pushed and forced into a structure to conform to the 'acceptable' ways of the world and our social communities, without identifying with our authentic selves first and our personal wants and needs.

Throughout the *Fourth* and *Fifth Agreements*, Don Miguel speaks of us being the masters of our own reality, and the creators of the dream of our lives, saying that:

*Every human is an artist. The dream of your life is to make beautiful art.*
*The dream you are living is your creation. It is your perception*

315

*of reality that you can change at any time. You have the power to create hell, and you have the power to create heaven. Why not dream a different dream? Why not use your mind, your imagination and your emotions to dream heaven?*

# Five Rules To Improve Your Life

Within the Five Agreements there are five specific lessons to assist us in understanding, coping, managing and bettering our lives. These agreements are:

1) BE IMPECCABLE WITH YOUR WORD

2) DON'T TAKE ANYTHING PERSONALLY

3) DON'T MAKE ASSUMPTIONS

4) ALWAYS DO YOUR BEST

5) BE SCEPTICAL, BUT LEARN TO LISTEN

*The only way to change your life is to change your choices, to change your actions.*

## Be Impeccable With Your Word

*Speak with integrity. Say only what you mean. Avoid using the word to speak against yourself or to gossip about others. Use your power of your word in the direction of truth and love.*

Being impeccable with your word starts with you; how you feel about yourself and the awareness of self. By being fully aware of your wants, needs and emotions, you are more likely to be able to control your reactions and therefore your words, using them in a positive light, rather than using them to hurt, blame or belittle someone else, or even yourself. Being impeccable with your word has a strong connection to Emotional Intelligence, especially regarding self-awareness and self-management. Having the ability to completely control how you speak and what you say, with truth and love, is a freeing and liberating way to live life that will only serve to benefit yourself and those around you.

Being impeccable with your word seems like an easy exercise; however, for many people it will cause them to be in uncomfortable situations for a number of reasons. For example, saying 'yes' and really meaning 'no' to a colleague, friend or acquaintance, or saying 'no' and setting personal boundaries, such as those in Emotional Intelligence and self-awareness. However, the more time you spend speaking your truth, the more inner freedom you will experience.

When you are impeccable with your word, you will feel good and be able to take responsibility for your actions, without any self-blame or judgement. Impeccability of the word-only improves our lives and will never be a destructive force towards anyone.

*You may have heard of the saying: 'a wise tongue is a still tongue'. This principle has similarities, though it goes so much further.*

## Don't Take Anything Personally

*Nothing other people do is because of you. It is because of themselves. All people live in their own dream, in their own mind; they are in a completely different world from the one we live in. When we take something personally, we make the assumption that they know what is in our world, and we try to impose our world on their world.*

This is absolutely true in life. Every single person looks at the world with a different perspective and vision. Where we are born, how we grow up, how we are educated, whether we have travelled, or not...etc., all have an effect on how we view the world. This means that another person's perspective of us is likely to be wildly different from our own.

As an example, if someone were to call you lazy. From their perspective you may be, even if you work 16 hours a day and work through the night. If they were to see you in bed at 10am, they may think you are lazy. Of course, they do not know the full facts of the situation, and this is the same with most people we will come into contact with throughout our lives.

We cannot take what someone else says about us personally, this is purely their own perspective and nothing to do with us. This is why it is crucial not to take anything personally; it is never anything to do with you, it is always another perspective.

When you do not take anything personally, you are able to live and speak your life without limitation, fear of ridicule or rejection from others. You will be able to open your heart fully and not be hurt by anyone's words or actions. By not taking anything personally you are giving yourself the gift of internal freedom, inner peace and liberation.

*There is a huge amount of freedom that comes to you when you take nothing personally.*

## Don't Make Assumptions

*All the sadness and drama you have lived in your life was rooted in making assumptions and taking things personally.*

Think about that sentence for a moment...all of the sadness and drama in life is caused by making assumptions and taking things personally. If we can teach ourselves to learn not to make assumptions, and not to take things personally, we will live a truly happy and contented life.

Making assumptions is something that most people do every day, and often every hour of every day. This could be as simple as assuming that your alarm clock will go off at the right time, assuming your partner knows you love them, assuming you will get a pay rise, assuming you have enough milk in the fridge for your breakfast...The problem we have in making assumptions is that we believe they are the truth, which creates unwanted or unrequired drama, pain and hurt.

Often, when we make assumptions, we are either afraid of what the truth may be or are comfortable with what we believe someone else is thinking. Neither scenario makes it possible, or probable, that you will have an accurate and successful outcome.

The best way to stop yourself from making assumptions is to be courageous, and to ask clear and concise questions until you have all the answers that you understand with clarity. If you are unsure of a response, ask for them to either repeat what they have said, or ask for another explanation so that you can understand clearly what they are describing to you.

*If we don't make assumptions, we can focus our attention on the truth, not on what we think is the truth. Then we see life the way it is, not the way we want to see it.*

## Always Do Your Best

*Doing your best is taking the action because you love it, not because you're expecting a reward. Most people do exactly the opposite: They only take action when they expect a reward, and they don't enjoy the action. And that's the reason why they don't do their best.*

It sounds pretty simple: always do your best. The real question is: how many of us do our best purely because we want to, and not for a reward? This is exactly what Daniel Goleman highlighted within his Emotional Intelligence, and motivation. When we do our best without expecting a reward, we are giving all we can so that we can fulfil our life's dreams and goals, which in turn will fulfil us through the achievement of our actions far more than any financial or monetary gains could do.

What Don Miguel Ruiz is suggesting is that when you do your best and give all you can, you will never look to the past and be critical of yourself that you could have done more, or that you could have spent more time working towards your goals and dreams.

When you do your best in any situation, it is not possible for you to judge yourself. Therefore, if you do not judge yourself then it is not possible for you to suffer from self-harm, fault or guilt. When you do your best and you can give no more, you will have no regrets in your actions. For if you, or someone else, were to judge you, you would be able to respond: 'I did all I could do, I could do no more,' and there would be no regrets.

*Just do your best – in any circumstance in your life. It doesn't matter if you are sick or tired, if you always do your best there is no way you can judge yourself. And if you don't judge yourself there is no way you are going to suffer from guilt, blame and self-punishment.*

## Be Sceptical, But Learn To Listen

*When you learn to listen, you know exactly what other people want. Once you know what they want, what you do with that information is up to you. You can react or not react, you can agree or disagree with what they say, and that depends on what you want.*

Listen but be sceptical. Ruiz says that most of what we hear is not truth, truth only becomes truth when we agree to what is said. Truth and fact are very different beings, someone can believe what they are saying is truth, whereas it could be littered with fictitious data or information. This is another reason why it is important for us not to make assumptions, and not to believe those assumptions, as when we do, we will not be speaking the truth.

Everything we say or do has been created by our own individual way of thinking and our own perspective, which has been created by our life experiences, our personalities, our education, our intelligence, our common sense…everything that anyone says or does is highly unlikely to be interpreted the same way as someone else.

This is where learning to listen, while remaining wary of what is said, is a key skill to master. Once you are able to understand the wants and needs of others, it becomes easier to accept, reject or just listen to the views and stories of what is being told to you at any given time.

*The fifth agreement is to be sceptical, but learn to listen. Be sceptical because most of what you hear isn't true. But the second half of the agreement is learn to listen, and the reason is simple: When you learn to listen, you understand the meaning of the symbols that people are using; you understand their story, and the communication improves a lot.*

## Don Miguel Ruiz's Final Say

Don Miguel Ruiz's books highlight some key skills that sit within Emotional Intelligence. They assist in you taking complete control of your life and ensuring that the decisions you make will only positively benefit you and your life.

### Do Not Fear To Live Your Best Life

*To be alive is the biggest fear humans have. Death is not the biggest fear we have; our biggest fear is taking the risk to be alive – the risk to be alive and express what we really are. Just being ourselves is the biggest fear of humans.*

### Living In The Moment Is The Only Way

*If you live in a past dream, you don't enjoy what is happening right now because you will always wish it to be different than it is. There is no time to miss anyone or anything because you are alive. Not enjoying what is happening right now is living in the past and being only half alive. This leads to self-pity, suffering and tears.*

### One More Day To Be Yourself

*The angel of death can teach us to live every day as if it is the last day of our lives, as if there may be no tomorrow. We can begin each day by saying, 'I am awake, I see the sun. I am going to give my gratitude to the sun and to everything and everyone, because I am still alive. One more day to be myself.'*

### Take Complete Control

*If you are impeccable with your word, if you don't take anything personally, if you don't make assumptions, if you always do your best, then you are going to have a beautiful life. You are going to control your life one hundred per cent.*

# The Power Of The Present Moment

*Realise deeply that the present moment is all you have. Make the NOW the primary focus of your life.*
Eckhart Tolle

# The Present Is The Only Gift You Need

*The Power of Now* by Eckhart Tolle is one of the most inspirational books in a generation, one that encapsulates the essence of being in the present moment, for it is the only moment that ever exists. Tolle says that, *'Nothing has happened in the past; it happened in the Now. Nothing will ever happen in the future; it will happen in the Now.'* It is for us to utilise the lessons within Emotional Intelligence, and for us to be self-aware enough to be in the present moment. Living each moment with freedom and peace.

The only moment in time that matters is the present moment, for, *'Life is now. There was never a time when your life was not now, nor will there ever be.'* When we are too focused on past events or our assumptions of the future, we lose sight of the now, and the now is the only place in time where anything ever happens. Every event, every feeling, every thought you have ever had has taken place in the now, in the present moment.

Time is a man-made creation that was devised to assist us in organising and structuring our lives by using the sun, stars and planetary movements. If you can imagine for a brief moment that you are able to speak with plants and animals, and were to ask a tree, a flower, a fish or a dog what the time or date was, they would all give you the same answer and say, *'The time is now. What else is there?'*

*Time isn't precious at all, because it is an illusion. What you perceive as precious is not time but the one point that is out of time: the Now. That is precious indeed. The more you are focused on time – past and future – the more you miss the Now, the most precious thing there is.*

Living life in the present moment will give you freedom from thought and freedom of life. Set yourself free.

## Do Not Live For Future Happiness, Be Happy Now

*It is not uncommon for people to spend their whole life waiting to start living.*

How many times have you thought about a moment in the future that you could not wait for? It could have been for a holiday, a wedding, the birth of a child, for a new job…etc. When we are in these moments, we almost run through life without living each day, living on autopilot until we get to our 'dream' situation. Then, it is usually on to the next.

By waiting and focusing your attention on future events, you are denying the present and rejecting all that it has to offer. Living in the present helps us to truly appreciate life; even if it is the smallest possible element, it can still be observed in the present and appreciated.

There is no need to wait for anything if you live in the present. Live your life like it is the last day you will have on Earth, and you will experience wonderful and liberating life changes.

## Do Not Fight The Present Moment, Welcome It As If It Was Your Choosing

*Accept – then act. Whatever the present moment contains, accept it as if you had chosen it. Always work with it, not against it. Make it your friend and ally, not your enemy. This will miraculously transform your whole life.*

What is in the present moment is reality, it is not your thoughts of what might be, or what you were expecting something to be, or not to be. The present moment only presents the truth, the reality of the situation, nothing more. Roll with it and go with the flow, the more you fight against the present, the more distress, upset and pain this can cause you. Accept the present moment, in all its glory, as if you had chosen it yourself.

## There Is No Regret, Stress and Sadness In The Now

*All negativity is caused by an accumulation of psychological time and denial of the present. Unease, anxiety, tension, stress, worry – all forms of fear – are caused by too much future, and not enough presence. Guilt, regret, resentment, grievances, sadness, bitterness, and all forms of non-forgiveness are caused by too much past, and not enough presence.*

With time being an illusion, a man-made creation to better the way in which we run our daily lives, our minds can be attached to the psychological time of past and future. If there is a situation in your past that did not go your way and you are still resisting that situation, you are also resisting the now and the truth, which causes self-pain and hurt. By denying a truth, especially one from the past, you will only harm yourself further. It is important to accept what is, for when you can accept, you will not punish and judge yourself any further.

## Living In The Past Will Harm Your Future

*If your mind carries a heavy burden of past, you will experience more of the same. The past perpetuates itself through lack of presence. The quality of your consciousness at this moment is what shapes the future.*

When we live in the past and hold onto the pain of the past, we are not only punishing ourselves further with that same pain and hurt previously experienced, we are ensuring our physical and mental memory retains this information for the continued use and abuse of ourselves. When you live in the present you will not be attacked by your mind, and the memories of past pain will subside. With careful self-reflection and self-management (EQ), in the future you will be left with a positive memory that you can emotionally control.

*Make peace with the past and live in the NOW.*

## Be In The Now And Be Free Of Negativity

*As soon as you honour the present moment, all unhappiness and struggle dissolves, and life begins to flow with joy and ease. When you act out the present-moment awareness, whatever you do becomes imbued with a sense of quality, care and love – even the simplest action.*

By keeping our minds in the present and not drifting off to past memories or future stresses we will be free of all the negative emotions that cause us disease and, in many cases, physical pain. All of our negative emotions come from either past events or future concerns, not in the present moment. Being emotionally self-aware, and in the moment, will ensure that you live a life that is free from self-emotional sabotage.

When you are in the present, there is only positivity and acceptance.

## Learn From Nature

*Watch any plant or animal and let it teach you acceptance of what is, surrender to the Now. Let it teach you Being. Let it teach you integrity – which means to be one, to be yourself, to be real. Let it teach you how to live and how to die, and how not to make living and dying into a problem.*

When we bring our attention to the natural world, and anything that has come to existence without the hand of human beings, we are transported out of the world of the mind and constant thought, and into a state of connectedness with Being, where everything in nature exists.

In bringing our mind to the attention of nature, it is not to simply think about a flower, tree, animal, rock...etc., it is to hold nature in our awareness, to be in the moment and a part of the moment. When you are fully aware in the moment, you will feel a state of Being and immense connection.

## Perception Is A Great Thing, It Is Never Real Life

*What a caterpillar calls the end of the world we call a butterfly.*

From a human perspective, watching a caterpillar transform into a butterfly is one of the most magical moments in nature. It is something to watch in awe. For the caterpillar, this could be one of the most terrifying and traumatic moments in their short life. It is only when the transformation is over that the butterfly can realise that it is not their death, but their birth.

It is important to remember that everything in our lifetimes happens for us and not to us. Every experience we encounter is there to help us learn a valuable lesson. Everything happens for a reason, whether we can understand the reason or not.

Accept what is reality and do not fight the truth.

## Live As If You Have Already Died

*The secret of life is to 'die before you die' – and find that there is no death.*

If you have ever had a moment when your life has been threatened, you will potentially be able to take this in more than someone who has not. When you experience a moment, or moments, when you are close to your physical end, you become very aware of life and living. This is something that we will all face at some point in our lives, we will all one day pass from this planet.

If you live your life as if it is the last day on earth, you would never live a dull day. You would appreciate everything and everyone around you. You would share your love, you would tell people how you really felt about them, you would be totally honest with everyone, including yourself. You would be completely and totally free.

# Eckhart Tolle: How Can You Be Present?

Using Eckhart Tolle's methods, I have outlined how you can take the initial steps to be present and find your Now. *'If you get the inside right, the outside will fall into place. Primary reality is within; secondary reality without.'*

## Surrender And Find Peace

*Don't look for peace. Don't look for any other state than the one you are in now; otherwise, you will set up inner conflict and unconscious resistance. Forgive yourself for not being at peace. The moment you completely accept your non-peace, your non-peace becomes transmuted into peace. Anything you accept fully will get you there, will take you into peace. This is the miracle of surrender.*

## Are You Being Present

*The moment you realise you are not present, you are present. Whenever you are able to observe your mind, you are no longer trapped in it. Another factor has come in, something that is not of the mind: the witnessing presence.*

To know that you are present, all you have to do is ask. Ask yourself: 'I am being present now?'

When you ask yourself, 'I am being present?' you return to the present moment, and see through *'present eyes'*. Look at what is around you, take in what you see, smell and feel. The bright and vivid colours, the clean, fresh smell of the air. Take it all in. Really feel it. Feel the energy. There is only positivity and calm in the present, where all darkness and confusion clears, giving rise to clarity and liberation.

Another extension of *'am I present?'* is to take all of your attention into the present by focusing on nature, a tree, a flower, an animal...etc. When you do this, notice the colours, the smells, the movement, or stillness in the moment. See the veins of the leaves, the shape of the petals, the animals living from the nectar and nutrients. Focus your attention on life – this is the very essence of NOW, and of BEING.

# Eckhart Tolle: The Key Take Away

## Take Action! You Will Either Win Or You Will Learn

*Any action is often better than no action, especially if you have been stuck in an unhappy situation for a long time. If it is a mistake, at least you learn something, in which case it's no longer a mistake. If you remain stuck, you learn nothing.*

## Three Lessons From Eckhart Tolle:

### *Life Is A Series Of Present Moments*

*The past is nothing more than all present moments that have gone by, and the future is just the collection of present moments waiting to arrive.*

### *All Negativity Is Caused From Denying The Present*

*All negativity is caused by an accumulation of psychological time and denial of the present.*

### *Stay In The Present And Be Free From Pain And Suffering*

*Nothing ever happened in the past that can prevent you from being present now, and if the past can't prevent you from being present now, what power does it have?*

*Realise deeply that the present moment is all you have. Make the NOW the primary focus of your life.*

# A Lighter And Brighter You

*Find your passion. Find your focus.*
*Free yourself, and have fun while doing it.*
Oliver Rolfe

# Deep Breathing And Meditation

This chapter has been edited with the assistance of Sara Leslie, international spiritual clairvoyant, medium and healer.

Deep breathing and meditation techniques and exercises take many forms and play an important role in assisting physical health, mental health, mindfulness and the metaphysical. Meditation is an important factor in many people's lives and seems to be everywhere around us, whether you live in the Eastern or the Western hemisphere. From Buddhist monks, to the most well-known and revered CEOs, celebrities and sportspeople on the planet. A vast number of people feel the benefits and personal development from meditation.

## Benefits Of Deep Breathing And Meditation

### *Feel Ageless And More Beautiful*

Breathing deeply slows the ageing process by increasing secretion of anti-aging hormones! By reducing stress, it improves your mood, elevating the levels of serotonin and endorphins.

### *Free Yourself From Pain*

When you deep breathe through meditation, the body releases endorphins, which are the feel-good hormones and a natural painkiller created by the body itself. It has also been said that deep breathing reduces inflammation in the body, due to the reduction of acid from having reduced stress in your life.

### *Feel Alive And Stay Safe*

When meditating on a regular basis your blood flow will increase, which means that you are getting more oxygen into your blood system. The result of this additional oxygen is increased energy levels. Additionally, increased oxygen levels also improve the body's immunity to outside viruses and bacteria.

## Take A Moment To Relax

Meditation is one of the most peaceful, relaxing and magical exercises anyone can achieve. With practice and patience, meditation can reset your mind, while you experience peace, calm and harmony all at once. German psychiatrist Johannes Heinrich Schultz developed a deep-breathing method of relaxation that is still one of the best-known Western relaxation techniques today. To enjoy a complete moment of calm…is to enjoy a moment of bliss.

## Improve Your Focus

There have been a number of studies undertaken globally, whereby the results all show that with regular deep breathing, your focus, attention and psychomotor functions all improve. When you meditate you stimulate the prefrontal cortex, this is the part of the brain responsible for concentration and problem-solving.

## Control Your Emotions

If you are ever overcome by emotion, being able to have control over your breathing will enable you to take steady, calm, deep breaths, bringing you back in control of yourself positively. With regular practice you can take control of your breath at will.

## Expand Your Memory

It has been found that with regular deep breathing, using a

technique called Deep Alternate-Nostril breathing, which has been traced back to a fifteenth-century manual on yoga by Swami Swatmarama, your memory recall can increase significantly.

## The Breathing Detox

When we breathe deeply, it helps the body to detoxify and release negative toxins that have been held in our bodily system. Studies undertaken by Michael Phillips of Menssana Research concluded that these toxins can include excess carbon dioxide, limonene, thymol, eucalyptol and sulphides. Additionally, when you breathe deeply on a regular basis, more oxygen will replace the negative toxins in your system.

## Calm Your Nerves And Ease Your Worries

Deep breathing or meditation exercises reduce stress and anxiety. Whether this is done regularly or at the time you need it most, being able to take 5-7 clear, slow, long, deep breaths will calm your nerves and give you a moment of clarity.

## Start On The Path To Enlightenment

Meditation can take many different forms, from simple deep breathing to the Buddhist monks seeking enlightenment. Meditation is something found in many, if not all, religions, in one form or another. This can include the reciting of prayers daily or the repetition of mantras. The goal is to achieve an altered state of consciousness with the intention of connection with a higher deity. The more time you can find for yourself to meditate, the more aware you will become of what your wants and needs truly are. What lies beneath, the true version of yourself. Regular meditation gives rise to clarity about what is important in life and a sense of confidence to make choices that ignite your passions and dissolve distractions. Suddenly a completely new world is opened to you, and it is totally different. Life takes on greater meaning and you feel a deeper sense of purpose and satisfaction.

# Deep Breathing And Meditation Exercises

Using my personal experiences, I have outlined a step-by-step guide to a simple deep breathing exercise and more detailed meditation to get you going. At this stage of the book, this is your opportunity to pause for a moment and work through an exercise at your own pace. Enjoy your moment and look forward to the peace, calm and serenity of meditation.

## Deep Breathing Exercise

*A Simple How-To Deep Breathing Guide*

- Either lying down, sitting or standing

- You can choose to open or close your eyes

- With your mouth closed

- Take a slow, steady inwards breath through your nose

- Allow your diaphragm and ribcage to expand as your lungs fill with air

- Once your lungs are fully expanded, hold for 3-5 seconds

- Exhale slowly through your mouth until you have no air left in your lungs

- Stop, and start again

- Continue this for 5-10 minutes, or as long as you feel you need

## Meditation Exercise

*A How-To Meditation Guide*

- Set some specific time aside to meditate, time just for you. Allow yourself a set amount of time (10-30 minutes to begin with).

- If you can have a fixed time daily or a weekly schedule, this will keep it clear for you and will help you look forward to this time.

- Before you begin, make sure you are comfortable.

- Wear comfortable clothing, nothing that will annoy, impede or irritate you. I would also suggest taking off rings, watches and bracelets as these can impede your clarity and cause distraction.

- It is a good idea to have some water nearby for before and after your meditation.

- Some people enjoy meditation music; if you do, now is the time to put it on (make sure it does not have adverts).

- Find a comfortable place to sit that is warm and where you will not be distracted. Somewhere you feel totally at ease and relaxed.

- It is possible to meditate in both low and natural light. Find what you feel most comfortable and relaxed with.

- Relax your body before you begin and let everything hang loose.

- Close your eyes and be aware of the space around you.

- Take a moment to notice the sounds, temperature, feeling of the room and how you feel.

- Clear your mind and set your intention for the meditation. Do you want to destress? Find an answer to a question? Take time for yourself?

- Say it three times in your mind.

- When you are ready to begin, take a long deep breath through your nose. All the while keeping your mouth closed.

- Allow your diaphragm and ribcage to expand as your lungs fill with air.

- Once your lungs are fully expanded, hold for 3-5 seconds.

- Exhale slowly through your mouth until you have no air left in your lungs.

- Stop, and start again.

- Do not worry about whether you are doing it 'the right way', look forward to this moment and focus only on your breathing.

- As you continue you will start to feel more relaxed.

- On your third or fourth breath, imagine that you have a beautiful warm beaming ray of light above your head.

- From now on, when you take in a breath see and feel that beautiful warm ray of light being breathed into your body. All the way from your head, right the way down to the ground through your toes.

- In this moment, you are able to assess your inner being. Realise that all is calm in this moment.

- At this time, you can send messages of positivity, health, success…to yourself from an altered, higher state.

- Imagine yourself in your future vision. Imagine yourself fully healthy, being promoted or having a family. Whatever you decide to choose at this time.

- Enjoy being in this moment.

- As you continue your breathing, be aware of your surroundings, of how you feel.

- When you feel that you are ready to end your meditation, start taking normal breaths.

- Start to bring your consciousness back to the room or space you are sitting in.

- Wiggle your fingers and toes to help bring yourself back to the room.

- When you feel alert and ready, open your eyes, giving yourself some time to adjust to the light.

- Take a drink of water to replenish yourself (staying hydrated is very important after a meditation).

- As soon as you have finished, stand up and move on with the day ahead, with great positivity.

# Johns Hopkins And NHS Breathing Techniques

Utilising the direct advice and guidance of Johns Hopkins Medicine and the NHS, I have included some important breathing techniques from these medical centres that will aid recovery from general lung problems, including COVID-19.

## Benefits Of Breathing Exercises

Peiting Lien, a clinical specialist at Johns Hopkins, believes that,

> Deep breathing can help restore diaphragm function and increase lung capacity. The goal is to build up the ability to breathe deeply during any activity, not just while at rest.

It is possible for anyone to benefit from deep breathing techniques and exercises, as they can lessen feelings of anxiety and stress, as well as improving sleep quality.

## Warning! Precautions

Do not begin exercises (and instead seek medical assistance) if:

- You have a fever
- You have any shortness of breath or difficulty breathing
- You have any chest pain or palpitations
- You have new swelling in your legs

STOP exercise immediately if you develop the following:

- Dizziness or excessive fatigue
- Shortness of breath (more than normal)

- Chest pain or irregular heartbeat
- Cool, clammy skin
- Any symptoms you consider an emergency

## Breathing Control

Breathing control is breathing gently to allow the airways to relax, using as little effort as possible. Breathing control can also help you when you are short of breath or feeling fearful, anxious or in a panic.

- Breathe in and out gently through your nose (if you can). If you find this difficult, breathe through your mouth instead.
- Breathe out through your mouth, purse your lips like you are blowing out a candle.
- Try to let go of any tension in your body with each breath out.
- Gradually try to make the breaths slower.
- Try closing your eyes to help you focus on your breathing and relax.

## Deep Diaphragmatic Breathing (Belly Breathing)

When we breathe deeply it helps to restore lung function by using the diaphragm. Breathing through the nose strengthens the diaphragm and encourages the nervous system to relax and restore itself.

When recovering from a respiratory illness, it is important not to rush recovery and put undue pressure on yourself. The following exercises can be conducted while laying on your back, sitting in a study chair or standing up, depending on your comfort and mobility levels.

- Place your hands around the sides of your stomach.
- Close your lips and place your tongue on the roof of your mouth.
- Breathe in through your nose (if you can) and pull the air down into your stomach where your hands are. Try to spread your fingers apart, in time with your breath.
- Slowly exhale your breath through your nose (if you can).
- Repeat deep breaths for one minute.

## *Humming*

Humming while exhaling helps increase nitric oxide production in the body. Nitric oxide helps with the building and repair of the nervous system, and it dilates blood vessels, enabling more oxygen to be delivered throughout the body. Humming can also assist in reducing stress, as it is calming and soothing.

- Sit upright on the edge of your bed or in a sturdy chair.
- Place your hands around the sides of your stomach.
- With your lips closed and your tongue on the roof of your mouth, breathe in through your nose and pull air down into your stomach where your hands are. Try to spread your fingers apart with your breath.
- Once your lungs are full, keep your lips closed and exhale while humming, making the 'hmmmmmm' sound. Notice how your hands lower back down.
- Again, inhale through your nose, then exhale through your nose while humming.
- Repeat for one minute.

# The Final Word

*You are the director of your life.*
*Be strong and live in the present moment.*
*Find your passion and take action today.*
Oliver Rolfe

# The Conclusion

So, we have now reached the end of this book and I hope that you have enjoyed the content; just as importantly, I hope that you have started to understand the underlying philosophy behind it.

We started by looking at the idea of 'Gestalt' (or wholeness) and suggested that it is vital to see yourself as a 'whole entity' when thinking about any self-improvement.

The book then went on to consider specific elements, such as your immune system, nutrition, mental health, energetic health, Emotional Intelligence, etc. Underpinning all of this is an appreciation that all of these facets are interlinked and entwined.

By keeping this in mind you will achieve a more 'total' transformation and learn to live not in the past, nor in the future, yet, in the HERE AND NOW!

# The Finale

Looking around there seems only confusion and madness. Here's to
the present moment, may it bring only gladness.

Do not look to the dark, but instead to light.
Never give up the hardest of fights.

Life is a journey for one and for all,
how you live it can make you stand tall.

Do not follow the crowd, instead, follow your feet.
Live your life to the sounds of your own heartbeat.

Your life can be tough, painful in places.
We accept what's been before us,
as this was G-d's graces.

On to the next, full of hope and belief.
Ahead full of promise and nothing but peace.

With family and team right by our side,
we promise to stand strong and never to hide.

With love and support giving strength to believe,
we know what must be done to follow our dreams.

We devote our lives to the ones we love,
with guidance and strength from the powers above.

To those that have wronged, it is never too late,
to put others first, and to save your own fate.

*Be no preacher, no Merlin, or no magician – we are one people, on our own solitary mission.*

*To one and to all, and to all a great year.*
*Go to the future with positivity, and with no fear.*

*Good luck in everything you do.*

*Be the best version of yourself.*

*Take Action Today!*

# Spartan International Group

## International Executive Recruitment And Life & Career/ Health & Wellbeing Consultancy

Should you wish to find out more details about our services, whether this is our Life & Career/Health & Wellbeing Coaching, looking for a career move or market/industry knowledge, please contact us.

**Website: www.spartan-int.com**

**Spartan Newsletter: https://spartanxtra.substack.com/**

**UK Phone: +44 203 372 5070**

**US Phone: +1 646 688 2393**

**Email: info@spartan-exec.com**

# Seminars And Workshops

To arrange more specific sessions based on the content of this book, contact us using the details below:

Use this reference when making contact:
**THE HOLISTIC GUIDE**

**Website: www.spartan-int.com**

**Spartan Xtra by Spartan International:
https://spartanxtra.substack.com/**

**UK Phone: +44 203 372 5070**

**US Phone: +1 646 688 2393**

**Email: info@spartan-exec.com**

# Video Guidance – Via YouTube

All of our videos are online now! Go to the Spartan International YouTube channel – Spartan Xtra by Spartan International for all our Life & Career/Health & Wellbeing videos…plus a couple of special editions.

**Spartan International YouTube Channel:**
https://www.youtube.com/channel/UCXUsiv0w74UZpsN9Ocl hy3w

Introduction – Welcome to Spartan Xtra:
https://www.youtube.com/watch?v=1DtNuWfb9Cs

*Body Language in Meetings – Part 1
https://youtu.be/D8mN2b0pGlM

*Body Language – Part 2
https://www.youtube.com/watch?v=rZoe9lzUX9o&t=234s

*Mindfulness and Mental Health
https://www.youtube.com/watch?v=jcUcefH2Mws

*Core Energy – How to Improve Yours
https://youtu.be/aXdzFRkJw1k

# Bibliography

For further reading of some of the key resources used in this book, please see below:

## It All Starts With You

Book:
*The Survivor's Guide to Your Career Today*
by Oliver Rolfe

Websites:
*https://www.glutenfreesociety.org/gluten-and-immune-system/*

*https://nutritionfacts.org*

*https://www.nccih.nih.gov/health*

*https://www.webmd.com/diet/*

*https://nutritiondata.self.com*

*https://www.healthline.com/nutrition*

*https://www.healthbenefitstimes.com*

*https://pubmed.ncbi.nlm.nih.gov/20146964/*

*https://www.health.harvard.edu/nutrition/why-nutritionists-are-crazy-about-nuts*

*https://ods.od.nih.gov/factsheets/list-all/*

*https://www.nhs.uk/conditions/vitamins-and-*

*minerals/https://www.webmd.com/vitamins/
index*

*https://medlineplus.gov/healthtopics.html*

## Mind Over Matter: A Matter Of The Mind

Books:          N/A

Websites:       *https://stepstogether.rehab*

*https://ourworldindata.org/mental-health*

*https://www.who.int/teams/mental-health-and-
substance-use/mental-health-in-the-workplace*

*https://www.nhsinform.scot/illnesses-and-
conditions/mental-health*

*https://www.ncbi.nlm.nih.gov/pmc/articles/
PMC1456909/*

*https://www.nhs.uk/oneyou/every-mind-matters/
possible-causes/*

*https://www.webmd.com/mental-health/mental-
health-causes-mental-illness##1*

*https://www.nccih.nih.gov/grants/mind-and-
body-research-information-for-researchers*

*https://pubmed.ncbi.nlm.nih.gov/18589562/*

*https://www.mentalhealth.org.uk/a-to-z/*

*p/physical-health-and-mental-health https:www. mind.org.uk/information-support/types-of mental-health-problems/mental-health-problems introduction/causes/*

*https://positivepsychology.com/mind-body-connection/*

## Feeling The Flow Of The Energy Within

Book:           *The Scientific Basis of Integrative Medicine* by Leonard A. Wisneski and Lucy Anderson

Websites:       *https://seventhlifepath.com/chakra-test/*

*https://www.researchgate.net/ publication/342562977_A_Brief_History_of_the_ Chakras_in_Human_Body*

*https://www.ncbi.nlm.nih.gov/pmc/articles/ PMC1142191/*

*https://www.mindbodygreen.com/0-91/The-7-Chakras-for-Beginners.html*

*https://www.soulfulcrystals.co.uk/chakra-balancing-crystals/*

*https://www.astralaspects.biz/shop/horoscopes/ chakras.html*

## Numbers Make The World Go Round

Books:       *Numerology – The Complete Guide, Volume 1*

by Matthew Oliver Goodwin

*Numerology – The Complete Guide, Volume 2*
by Matthew Oliver Goodwin

*The Secret Science of Numerology*
by Shirley Blackwell Lawrence

*Numerology, an Idiot's Guide*
by Jean Simpson

*Numerology*
by Michelle Buchanan

*Chaldean Numerology – For Beginners*
by Heather Alicia Lagan

Websites:     *https://www.tsemrinpoche.com/tsem-tulku-rinpoche/numerology/numerology-calculator.html?gclid=EAIaIQobChMIvNmZxvGf6gIVV-DtCh0ULAUNEAAYASAAEgIpePD_BwE*

*https://numerologist.com*

*https://www.psychics4today.com/numerology-numbers-and-meanings/*

*https://annperrynumerologist.com*

## Numbers: The Universal Language

Books:     *Angel Numbers*
by Doreen Virtue

*Angel Numbers*
by Kyle Gray

Websites:     *https://www.mirrorhour.com*

*http://sacredscribesangelnumbers.blogspot.
com/p/what-are-angel-numbers.html*

*http://sacredscribesangelnumbers.blogspot.
com/p/index-numbers.html*

## Emotional Intelligence: The Key To Understanding Who We Are

Books/Articles:   *Emotional Intelligence*
by Daniel Goleman

*What Makes a Leader?*
by Daniel Goleman

Primal Leadership: The Hidden Driver of
Great Performance
by Daniel Goleman, Richard Boyatzis and
Annie McKee

Websites:     *https://online.hbs.edu/blog/post/emotional-
intelligence-in-leadership*

*https://www.talentsmart.com/about/emotional-
intelligence.php*

*https://hbr.org/2018/10/working-with-people-
who-arent-self-aware*
*https://www.maetrix.com.au/emotional-*

*intelligence/*

*https://virtualspeech.com/blog/5-features-emotional-intelligence*

*https://www.healthline.com/health/emotional-intelligence#components*

*https://positivepsychology.com/emotional-intelligence-eq/*

*https://hbr.org/2015/03/research-were-not-very-self-aware-especially-at-work*

*https://dougbelshaw.com/blog/2009/07/01/daniel-goleman-on-leadership-and-emotional-intelligence/*

## Advanced Body Talk – The Unspoken Language

Book:    *The Dictionary of Body Language – A Field Guide to Human Behaviour*
by Joe Navarro

Websites:    N/A

## Blink: Seeing Is Really Believing

Book:    *Blink*
by Malcolm Gladwell

Websites:    N/A

## The Five Cornerstones Of A Controlled, Happy And Contented Life

Books:
*The Four Agreements*
by Don Miguel Ruiz

*The Fifth Agreement*
by Don Miguel Ruiz and Don Jose Ruiz

Website:
*https://www.thefouragreements.com*

## The Power Of The Present Moment

Books:
*The Power of Now*
by Eckhart Tolle

*Practising The Power of Now*
by Eckhart Tolle

Websites:
N/A

## A Lighter And Brighter You

Book:
*The Survivor's Guide to Your Career Today*
by Oliver Rolfe

Websites:
*https://enderley.nhs.uk/wp-content/uploads/2020/04/Covid-booklet-post-discharge-hospital-FINAL.pdf*

*https://www.hopkinsmedicine.org/health/conditions-and-diseases/coronavirus/coronavirus-recovery-breathing-exercises*

# Disclaimer

This book is presented solely for educational, motivational and entertainment purposes. The author and publisher are not offering it as legal, psychological or other professional services advice. While best efforts have been used in preparing this book, the author and publisher make no representations or warranties of any kind and assume no liabilities of any kind with respect to the accuracy or completeness of the contents and specifically disclaim any implied warranties of merchantability or fitness of use for a particular purpose. Neither the publisher nor the author shall be liable for any physical, psychological, emotional, financial, or commercial damages, including, but not limited to, special, incidental, consequential or other damages or be responsible to any person or entity with respect to any loss or incidental or consequential damages caused, or alleged to have been caused, directly or indirectly, by the information or programmes contained herein. No warranty may be created or extended by sales representatives or written sales materials. Every company is different and the advice and strategies contained herein may not be suitable for your situation. You should seek the services of a competent professional before beginning any improvement programme. Our views and rights are the same: You are responsible for your own choices, actions and results.

YOUR HEALTH, YOUR LIFE, YOUR DECISION

# Notes

# Notes

# Notes

# Notes

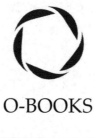

# O-BOOKS

# SPIRITUALITY

O is a symbol of the world, of oneness and unity; this eye represents knowledge and insight. We publish titles on general spirituality and living a spiritual life. We aim to inform and help you on your own journey in this life.
If you have enjoyed this book, why not tell other readers by posting a review on your preferred book site?

## Recent bestsellers from O-Books are:

### Heart of Tantric Sex
Diana Richardson
Revealing Eastern secrets of deep love and intimacy to Western couples.
Paperback: 978-1-90381-637-0 ebook: 978-1-84694-637-0

### Crystal Prescriptions
The A-Z guide to over 1,200 symptoms and their healing crystals
Judy Hall
The first in the popular series of eight books, this handy little guide is packed as tight as a pill-bottle with crystal remedies for ailments.
Paperback: 978-1-90504-740-6 ebook: 978-1-84694-629-5

## Take Me To Truth
Undoing the Ego
Nouk Sanchez, Tomas Vieira
The best-selling step-by-step book on shedding the Ego, using the teachings of *A Course In Miracles*.
Paperback: 978-1-84694-050-7 ebook: 978-1-84694-654-7

## The 7 Myths about Love...Actually!
The Journey from your HEAD to the HEART of your SOUL
Mike George
Smashes all the myths about LOVE.
Paperback: 978-1-84694-288-4 ebook: 978-1-84694-682-0

## The Holy Spirit's Interpretation of the New Testament
A Course in Understanding and Acceptance
Regina Dawn Akers
Following on from the strength of *A Course In Miracles*, NTI teaches us how to experience the love and oneness of God.
Paperback: 978-1-84694-085-9 ebook: 978-1-78099-083-5

Readers of ebooks can buy or view any of these bestsellers by clicking on the live link in the title. Most titles are published in paperback and as an ebook. Paperbacks are available in traditional bookshops. Both print and ebook formats are available online.
Find more titles and sign up to our readers' newsletter at
http://www.johnhuntpublishing.com/mind-body-spirit
Follow us on Facebook at https://www.facebook.com/OBooks/
and Twitter at https://twitter.com/obooks